Jennifer's Way

Jennifer's Way

my journey with celiac disease—
what doctors don't tell you
and how you can
learn to live again

Jennifer Esposito

with Eve Adamson

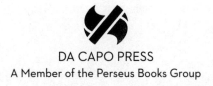

DA CAPO PRESS
A Member of the Perseus Books Group

Printed in the United States of America.

For information, address Da Capo Press, 44 Farnsworth Street, 3rd Floor, Boston, MA 02210.

Set in 12 point Adobe Garamond by Marcovaldo Productions, Inc., for the Perseus Books Group

Cataloging-in-Publication data for this book is available from the Library of Congress.
First Da Capo Press edition 2014
ISBN: 978-0-7382-1710-9 (Hardcover)
ISBN: 978-0-7382-1711-6 (eBook)

Published by Da Capo Press
A Member of the Perseus Books Group
www.dacapopress.com

Da Capo Press books are available at special discounts for bulk purchases in the U.S. by corporations, institutions, and other organizations. For more information, please contact the Special Markets Department at the Perseus Books Group, 2300 Chestnut Street, Suite 200, Philadelphia, PA, 19103, or call (800) 810-4145, ext. 5000, or e-mail special.markets@ perseusbooks.com.

10 9 8 7 6 5 4 3 2 1

This book is dedicated to every celiac,
whether diagnosed or not.
I hope this book gives you some understanding and peace.
I thank this community from the bottom of my heart.
You were the first to help me understand this new world.

contents

two   *Your Journey*

foreword

By Patrick Fratellone, M.D.

The last patient of the day on a cold December evening was Jennifer Esposito. I had never seen her Academy Award–winning film, *Crash*, but I had seen the popular Friday night show, *Blue Bloods*. Yet, the woman sitting there in front of me seemed to have no correlation to the vibrant character she played on TV. This woman was distressed, unkempt, and suffering on all levels. Her chief complaint on the intake form read: *Overall poor health*. She wrote that she suffered from daily headaches with a severity of 7 to 8 on a scale of 10. Under "duration" she had written: *For years—getting worse*.

When she came to see me, Jennifer had already been diagnosed with celiac disease by biopsy as well as serum blood testing. She had been on a quest to remain 100% gluten free, but she was still having many health issues. She had suffered since childhood, and I wondered, as I listened to her story, how she had survived all these years. Clearly she was determined, and was highly motivated to understand her disease. I could relate to that—I have celiac disease, too, and it took me a long time to get diagnosed. Once I was, I wanted to know everything, just as she did. When I was diagnosed, nobody said anything about diet.

I explained to Jennifer that celiac disease is an autoimmune disease, and is often accompanied by other autoimmune diseases. She might well have some other condition that had yet to be diagnosed. I drew her a diagram of the small intestine that looked like a shag carpet. I explained that this protein, gluten, had flattened that carpet into a Berber rug. The small intestine is essential for the absorption of nutrients, the production of vitamin D3, and crucially, the manufacture of the neurotransmitter, serotonin. When serotonin is low, the body overproduces norepinephrine, which can cause severe anxiety. This process also depresses GABA production, which can cause sleep disturbance.

As I spoke, tears welled in her eyes and then she began to cry. The emotional impact of finally being heard by a doctor was overwhelming to her. We discussed food rotation as a way to take her gluten-free diet and make it even safer for her delicate system. We discussed the "energy thieves" in her life that were making her condition worse—stress, overwork, anxiety. We discussed meditation and prayer. I began to paint a picture of the woman she would become as we wrestled down her celiac disease.

Today, I see a different Jennifer Esposito. She is not without health issues. Managing her disease is her daily duty, but she takes the job very seriously, and it shows. She has reclaimed a vibrancy she once had, and she is living a life that works. She has a purpose, and the energy she needs to fulfill it. She may not get to eat or even feel like someone who doesn't have celiac disease, but she gets to feel like herself. She is alive, inspired, and is reaching out to help others, through her blog, her bakery, and now, through this book. It has been a beautiful evolution to witness—from darkness, in the place she was when we first met, back into the light of her own purpose and promise.

I am proud and privileged to be part of her life, and to have played a small part in her discovery of her own "new normal." She has taught me much over the years, which reminds me of the William Osler quote, "Medicine is not taught in the classroom, but at the bedside." May this book teach you much as well, giving you the insight and the inspiration to take back your own life from the grip of celiac disease and learn how to live again.

—*Patrick Fratellone, M.D.*

introduction

Being an actress and in the public eye for almost twenty years, I can count on one hand the number of times I've been in the press for anything other than promoting the project of the moment. If you had told me years ago that I would write a book so openly about my personal life, I would have said you were crazy.

When I was diagnosed with celiac disease, all that changed and I felt almost compelled to tell my story. This disease has taken many twists and turns and has been at the root of many unanswered questions in my life since I was a child. The pain and suffering, not only physical but emotional, is something I wish on no one. If there is one paragraph, even just one sentence in this book that helps you in any way to understand what may be going on in your life with your health, then that is what I set out to do.

I believe there are a few very basic needs for us, as human beings. We want to feel safe, loved, accepted, and heard. Most if not all people with celiac disease are threatened in a big way. Feeling safe becomes something that doesn't apply to you anymore. You are not just in the hands of doctors who are often not able to tell you what's wrong—for most people, an accurate diagnosis takes years—but you are also at the mercy of every meal. Food becomes an enemy that you must keep your eye on at all times. Feeling loved gets threatened when family, friends, and society don't really get this disease, or at least not fully, or not yet. That can be very isolating at times, leaving people feeling unloved.

That brings me to acceptance. Everyone wants to feel a part of something. Not being able to conduct your life as everyone else does is not only hard on the social aspect of your life, but on your heart as well.

Finally, that leads me to the last basic human need, and to be honest, this has been the biggest single reason I have opened my life up and related my struggles to you: so you can feel like you can tell your story and be heard. I take you all the way back through my childhood, in the hopes that you will see in my early symptoms clues to help you understand yours. I want to show you by example that not all celiac disease symptoms are stomach-related, and some symptoms can seem far-removed from your gut. I take you even further back, showing you that my mother and grandmother had symptoms, too, to show you that celiac disease can be passed along through families for generations, so you can look back at your own family history for clues and validation. When I finally found out I had celiac disease, I realized how far back it went.

My ultimate intention in telling this story is to help you find your voice. I cannot count the number of people who have written to me and come in to my bakery from around the world, just to say *thank you for telling my story by telling yours.* I want to give a voice and a face to this disease. Many people have been unheard for so long regarding this disease, as I was. Some were told they were crazy, some given a wrong diagnosis, and many are still searching for an answer. This leaves people feeling unheard, and as I say in the first chapter in this book, it is my experience that something happens to you when you go for so long without being heard. Your soul starts to die a little. You stop voicing your opinions and concerns, your gut stops speaking to you, and you become someone who doesn't believe their words matter.

If I say anything in this book that you hear, please hear this: *your voice matters and your symptoms are real and there are people out there who will listen. You can be heard and you will be heard.* I am here to tell you that I get it. I hear you.

one

My Journey

1

80 degrees and sunny

I hadn't noticed the weather that day. I hadn't noticed the sun, the heat, the blue sky—the only thing I noticed was my illness. It had overtaken me to the point where there was no seeing—not the weather, not my family, not my life.

I'd been getting recurring, extreme sinus infections every couple of months, then every couple of weeks, then week after week. I'd been taking antibiotics for months to try to get ahead of the infections, but they weren't working. Then I noticed the large lump on my neck. Was it cancer? I was sure it had to be cancer. Why else would I feel like I was dying?

Finally, my ENT gave up. "I don't know what this is anymore," he told me, holding out his hands. "I want you to see this general practitioner." He handed me a name scrawled on a card. "She's good. Maybe she can figure out what's going on."

I had all but given up, too. I was so ill, I didn't have the energy to fight anymore. After years of constant illness, I'd stopped trying to figure out what was wrong with me. I just wanted someone to tell me the answer, to say, "Jennifer, you have X." Even if it was a death sentence, I didn't care. I would be psyched, just to *know.* I'd tried everything I could think of. And now I was done.

But I was a good patient, so I made an appointment with the GP. She sat with me for about an hour, asking me all the questions I'd been asked before by a hundred other doctors. I answered mechanically, without expression. I'd lost faith in doctors by this point. I felt so completely and utterly ill that I had nothing left to give beyond my memorized litany of unexplained symptoms: Sleeping close to thirteen hours a night and waking up exhausted, constant stomach problems, raging panic attacks, joint pain, buckling knees, extreme weakness, yellowing skin, painful canker sores, excruciating sinus headaches, numbness, tingling, and hair and nails so weak they broke off at the slightest pressure—not to mention the huge lump now protruding from my neck, just under my ear.

The doctor asked me question after question, expressionless as she wrote down what I said. And then, of course, came the questions about my family history—my mother's chronic illnesses, panic attacks, depression. My grandmother's stomach issues and death from cancer. Had I traveled out of the country? Had I been exposed to anything? Did I work around toxic products? Was I stressed? *Of course I'm stressed,* I wanted to scream. *I've been sick for as long as I can remember and I just want someone to figure out why!* But I didn't have the energy to scream. I answered the questions, as calmly and rationally as I could, even though I was trembling all over, from the inside out, vibrating with anxiety, pain, and exhaustion.

Every new specialist, every new theory, every new appointment, even every new symptom had triggered the false hope that finally I had the key to the a-ha moment I'd been waiting for—a real diagnosis. But it had never come, and now I feared it never would. Earlier that week, a tooth had literally come flying out of my mouth. Something was seriously wrong with me. Teeth don't just fall out for no reason. Lumps don't just form for no reason. But nobody knew the reason, and now I just wanted to close my eyes, curl up in a ball, and have it all be over. Next, it was time for the physical exam. She took me into the exam room and I could barely climb onto the exam table. She checked my pulse, took my temperature, and ran her hands around my body, lingering over the lump on my neck. She was very quiet and calm as she listened to my heartbeat. She wrote some things down on the chart, took a beat, removed her stethoscope, and gently put her hand on my slumped back. My body stiffened at her touch, then melted from exhaustion, but her quiet confidence made me wonder: Had she found it? Was it something in plain sight the others had missed? I couldn't bear to be disappointed again, but what if…

She cleared her throat. I looked up. I actually managed to smile in the face of my impending diagnosis. She smiled back sadly and said, "Jennifer, do you want to kill yourself?"

My face fell. I stared at her. I had no words. Is that how I looked to her? Suicidal? I couldn't believe that of all the things she could have said, this is what she felt she needed to ask me. Sure, I was depressed. Who wouldn't be depressed, being sick *all the damn time?* I was afraid I was going to die, but I certainly didn't want to kill myself.

Tears began to roll down my cheeks, and I feared they might confirm her suspicions, but I had nothing left inside with which to defend myself. I knew that even with years of debilitating symptoms, I had managed to become a self-made, hard-working, award-winning actress, that I had owned my own home by the age of twenty-five, that I was a good friend, a doting aunt, a devoted godmother, a loyal sister, and a self-respecting thirty-five-year-old woman. I knew I'd traveled all over the world by myself, had good relationships and bad, that I had cried, learned, pulled myself back up. I knew that I worked out and never took a recreational drug in my life, that I loved food and travel and my family and my *life.* I knew I meditated and had a strong spiritual center, and that I'd been in very low places, but always counted my blessings rather than focusing on what I didn't have. *I knew how much I had to live for.* Couldn't she see that?

But I couldn't seem to muster a single word. I was devastated, sick, so tired I could barely sit upright—no wonder she thought I was suicidal. And her question begged another one: What if my symptoms weren't real? What if it was all in my head? Was I making myself sick? Was I actually mentally, rather than physically, ill?

I knew it wasn't true. The tooth, the lump, the decades of pain, it was all real. And yet, doctor after doctor had offered me not a diagnosis, not an answer, but antidepressants, Valium, Ativan, Klonopin, enough to start a small drug ring (or at least a pharmacy). And why? Because the colonoscopies, barium enemas, MRIs, CT scans, X-rays, nerve tests, and too many vials of blood taken had all shown nothing. I'd been given physical diagnoses, usually vague ones that really meant, "We don't know what's wrong with you"—Epstein-Barr virus, irritable bowel syndrome, chronic fatigue. I'd been treated for a phantom parasite that was never actually found, tested for MS, lupus, Lyme disease, hepatitis, rheumatoid arthritis, and more. After every test, I always got that *look*. That "it might just be in your head" look. And then, the prescriptions and the referral to the therapist. Always the therapist. Always the implication: "What you really need, lady, is a shrink."

I couldn't do it anymore. I was so tired of explaining and begging people to help me, of being ignored, disregarded, and undermined. Inside my head, I was screaming: *I'm not crazy! I'm not suicidal! Please don't send me away with another prescription for Valium and the number of your favorite psychiatrist! I don't need antidepressants! I need help!*

But she was waiting for answer. I needed to focus. Her question reverberated: "Jennifer, do you want to kill yourself?" All I could do was shake my head. And then, from somewhere within, the words emerged—a last desperate attempt. A distress call, an SOS rising out of the storm that was made of the tears raining down my face and dripping from my chin. Almost without realizing I was speaking, I heard myself say, in a voice that was small and vulnerable and nothing like how I used to think of myself: "I need help. Please. Help me."

I was begging for my life with what felt like my last breath. I laid it all at her feet. I looked her in the eyes and she looked back.

Then she put her hand on my trembling hand, and said, with a sincerity I hadn't heard from a doctor before, "Okay. I'll find out what's wrong."

THE NEXT DAY, I woke up in the morning after a full night's sleep, totally exhausted, again. As I lay there, trying to find the energy to get out of bed, not yet willing to deal with the day, I kept hearing the doctor's voice. "Jennifer, do you want to kill yourself?" The words ran over and over in my head like a recording on a loop. The way she had said it was loving, almost kind. I couldn't help wondering: Was she right? Did she see something I didn't see? Had I given up? The notion calmed me. Maybe it *was* all in my head, after all. Deep down in my heart, I didn't believe it. My symptoms were too tangible. But wouldn't it be so much easier to just give up and accept what everyone was telling me? What if I just said "Okay," and stopped fighting? What if I just accepted the pain in my joints and the burning in my stomach and the anxiety that wracked my every move? What if I just took whatever drug of the week they wanted to give me and let it be? A tear rolled off my face and on to my pillow. Whatever this doctor told me, I decided, would be my final destination. Even if she told me I was crazy.

Suddenly, a bump on the bed jolted me out of my thoughts. I looked down to see two smiling faces and wagging tails. Frankie Bean, my Golden Retriever, and Betty Boop, my Bernese Mountain Dog. My two big goofy pups, who always knew when I was upset, who always tried to comfort me. Frankie Bean pushed his nose under my hand. Betty Boop woofed in her gentle way. They snuggled up to me, burrowing their wet noses into the space between my neck and the pillow, forcing their panting, grinning heads under my hands for petting.

"Hi pups," I said, patting them both. I knew they would love a walk, but those days I could barely make it to the door so they could go out and do their business. I'd missed so much because of my health. Dinner parties I'd skipped because of stomach problems, invitation lists I'd been removed from by former friends and important business people because I'd cancelled on them one too many times. Appointments missed or never scheduled because I was never sure I would be able to make them. In fact, a pretty big chunk of my life revolved around planning for my symptoms and the havoc they wreaked on my life. It was no way to live.

"That's it," I thought. I reached for the phone to call the doctor and ask for the medication she had prescribed during my appointment that I hadn't accepted. Then I realized it was Sunday. It would have to wait another day. Sunday meant something, though. It meant Agape.

If I was planning to go anywhere or do anything today, maybe Agape was the answer. Agape is a church in Los Angeles that had helped me through some pretty rough times in my life. It is a community of pure positivity, with the overall message that if you let things be, if you accept reality with gratitude, then you can finally find peace. That sounded like just what I needed. I needed to accept my fate, my unexplained symptoms, the idea that it was all in my head. I would take their drugs. I would let her think I was suicidal. If I'm nuts, then so be it. Got the message, doc. It's not you, it's me. It sounded wrong in my heart, but what else could I do? I was waving the white flag. Acceptance. Yes.

Although I could barely stand, my knees giving out, weakness overwhelming me, panic always brewing in my chest like an incoming storm, although I was barely functioning as a human being any-more, I would get up and get to Agape somehow. It was a last-ditch effort to survive, going to the only place I knew that might be in line with my need to accept my circumstances. I would do it, if not for me, then for my pups, who needed me to take them for walks again. If this was to be my new way of life, I was going to have to deal with it. It was the only option I could think of besides never getting out of bed again.

I summoned all the strength I had left to get up, get dressed, wash my face, and put on blush to cover my sallow, ashen complex-ion. I brushed my hair and tried to ignore the strands coming out by the brush-full. I picked up my car keys, kissed my pups, and hobbled out to the car. Once I was on the road, I opened all the windows, trying to invigorate myself and give myself the energy to get there. The air actually felt good on my skin, a sensation I hadn't felt in awhile. I'd been housebound for days.

As I got on the 405, I noticed the silence. It was early, so there weren't many cars on the road. I liked that silence, so I didn't turn on the radio the way I usually did. I drove this way for awhile, just me and my thoughts. Then my phone rang, jangling through the Bluetooth hands-free connection on my car. I pressed the button on the steering wheel.

"Hello?"

"Hi. How have you been?" My older sister's voice crackled through the speakers. "Are you feeling any better?"

I sighed. "No," I said. I began to tell her about the last couple of days, when I noticed a flatbed truck in front of me with a large amount of wood piled precariously on top. I didn't think much about it beyond a passing thought that it looked like a hazard. I slowed down a bit, to put some distance between myself and the truck, and began to tell my sister about my most recent decision: To give up. To just accept that I would never get a diagnosis. To just do whatever the doctor said. "I can't do it anymore," I said.

"I'm going to just take whatever they tell me to take, even if they say it's all in my…"

BOOM. A sound like a cannon, the splintering crack of glass, white light—at that exact moment, just as I spoke those words, a 4x6 piece of wood from that flatbed truck had come hurtling through my windshield, stopping just inches from my face, then swinging around, hitting my rearview mirror, and falling into my lap, along with chunks of glass, then bouncing up to hit the sunroof. Glass rained down on my head as my car skidded and swerved. I screamed, and my sister screamed, too, hearing the whole thing over the phone, and then we were disconnected, and everything was silent. My car sat, half on and half off the shoulder, crushed and shattered. The flatbed truck drove on, oblivious to its role in my near destruction.

I sat there in shock, covered in glass, staring at that huge chunk of wood. I was afraid to move because of all the glass. Slowly, carefully, I picked up my phone and dialed 911, and then my assistant, Jackie. My hands and arms were covered in tiny little cuts, some filling up with blood. I looked up at the cars zooming by. Surely, somebody would stop to see if the driver was okay. I wasn't even sure whether I was okay or not. I was paralyzed and numb. I watched them pass, car after car, on their way to somewhere else, everyone inexplicably in a hurry on a Sunday morning.

Nobody stopped. Not one car. Not one person pulled over to help me. I was a girl in a car on the side of the road, covered in glass and blood, but the world kept spinning. I waited for help, stunned and terrified. I waited and waited. I sobbed, but tried not to move, terrified that anything I did might drive those shards of glass further into my skin. No one came for what seemed like hours.

As I sat there on that gorgeous California day, I felt invisible, as if my desperation had erased me from the radar of humanity. I realized just how long I had been waiting for help of every kind: help from doctors, agents, managers, strangers on the road. Help from medicine, and now from 911. It took them 25 minutes to get to me. Why was it so hard to get help? Why wasn't anyone listening? And what was the lesson? My mind kept drifting to this last question, as I sat there dazed and alone. What was I supposed to make of all this?

I've always believed that every experience has a lesson, and I've always believed in signs. This seemed like a giant billboard of a sign, but what did it say? Was it a sign that no one cared? To have faith? But in what? I looked around me. I was totally alone and even though I was covered in broken glass, a sense of calm came over me. I was slipping into survival mode. I think it happens to anyone who experiences a trauma. I felt it click in, and I realized: I had to have faith in myself. I had to help myself. That 4x6 came at me just at the moment when I was ready to give up, to accept that my intuition was wrong and that the doctors must be right. Maybe God or the universe or whatever it is that guides us was sending me a loud-and-clear message: To have faith in myself, my instincts, and what my heart has been telling me all along. Faith that no matter what anybody else says, I was going to have to find the answers myself. I was literally and metaphorically alone in this, but that doesn't make me wrong. It's my life and my health, and nobody understands it like me. I knew there was something wrong with me, and no matter if this doctor or that doctor or the tenth doctor down the line doesn't see it. Somebody would, but it was up to me to make it happen. I was ready to give up, but now I saw that I couldn't give up. Not now. Not ever.

The EMTs looked me over and told me to go home and get in the shower to loosen any leftover pieces of glass from my hair and skin. Jackie put me in her car, told me how lucky I was to be alive, and drove me home. I felt a lot of things at the moment, but lucky was not exactly one of them. Later, after a long day of friends calling, dealing with the insurance company, rental cars, and the seemingly endless process of dislodging bits of glass from the most unlikely places, I finally stopped shaking. I lay down on my bed, in anticipation of the doctor's call in the morning. I knew that whatever she said, I would stop at nothing to get an answer. I closed my eyes.

THE NEXT MORNING, the phone rang. It was Dr. Mendel. "Jennifer," she said, in her warm voice. "I have an answer. I know exactly what's wrong with you."

I held my breath. I waited. Was it impending death? Or was it life?

"You have celiac disease. The worst case I've ever seen."

Celiac disease? I had absolutely no idea what she was talking about.

2

hungry

*n*early ten pounds, with jet-black hair and tremendous cheeks, I began life with an allergic reaction. Covered head to toe with a terrible rash, I was diagnosed with an allergy to the soap I was washed in at birth. My mother called me her little pink butterball because of my rashy cheeks, and when the nurses refused to let her hold me and dress me (in the early 1970s, mothers weren't trusted with their own newborns), she demanded they hand me over.

There were many clues that my health was off, right from the beginning—clues easily misinterpreted as proof that I was a good, robust, healthy child, but which actually hinted at something more insidious to come. First and foremost was the one thing that defined my childhood: my constant, insatiable, unrelenting hunger. My mother tells me that, as a baby, she had to feed me with both hands. One hand with a spoonful of food was going in while the other hand had a second spoonful coming in right behind it. That second spoonful had to be there or I wouldn't let the first spoon out of my mouth! Nothing made me angrier than the end of a meal. I screamed my head off every time.

I loved food. I've always loved food. It's an intimate part of who I am. Maybe it's my Italian heritage, or maybe it's just me, but food has always meant love, belonging, connection, pleasure, and joy. I know some people don't care all that much about food, but I can't imagine what that would be like. I live for the smells, the tastes, the textures, and the context of good food and a good meal. To me, it is one of the most important parts of life.

Most of my earliest memories involve food in some capacity: Climbing up the cabinets to get to the pancake mix, to make breakfast for my sleeping family, when I was only five years old. Slumber parties with my cousin that primarily centered around hiding food under our makeshift tent in her bedroom, then gorging on it all night long. The Sunday feasts with my family involved course after course of pure joy. One of my favorite memories is walking with my dad to the corner bakery on the weekends in Brooklyn to buy fresh jelly doughnuts, onion rolls, bagels, and rainbow cookies. The savory-sweet aroma that wafted over me as we stepped up to the counter almost made me swoon in intoxication from sugar and happiness. Then it was on to the deli for white fish, lunchmeats, and my favorite: a sleeve of Oreos that my father and I shared on the walk home, without telling my mother. Our food forays were the best times I ever had with my father.

But it wasn't all decadence. My mother had strict rules about the foods we were allowed to have (hence the sneaking of the Oreos). Our house contained no sugary cereals, no candy, and no soda. On the weekdays, oatmeal was my breakfast. My older sister of seven years, Suzanne, sat next to me at the table in protest. She said the oatmeal was slimy. She was a god to me back then, so I protested right along with her, but secretly, even oatmeal was a feast. After my sister left the table, I always asked for seconds. I loved the warm comforting oats with milk and brown sugar.

But oatmeal couldn't compare to the breakfast my father made on the weekends. After our trek to the bakery for jelly doughnuts, my father made "dunked eggies," an over-easy egg served with a warm onion roll smothered in fresh sweet butter. I pinched off bits of bread with my fingers and dunked them into the warm egg yolk. The taste of the onion, bread, salty butter, thick savory yolk—it was magic to me.

Weekends were the best. When it was time for lunch, my dad and I broke out all the cold cuts we bought and made submarine sandwiches filled with ham, salami, cheese, sweet peppers, and mustard. If it was Sunday, however, we saved our appetites for a dinner of macaroni and meatballs, one of my all-time favorite things. I drowned every strand of pasta with tons of Parmigiano cheese so that every bite was full of tender pasta, warm sauce, and tangy melting cheese.

But even that dinner was a distant second to what we ate on our outings to L&B Spumoni Gardens Pizza in Bensonhurst or Nathan's Hot Dogs in Coney Island. The whole family piled into the car and headed out, eager to eat our faces off! L&B Spumoni Gardens is eighty years old, and to this day, I believe it makes one of the best pizzas I've ever had the good fortune to taste. As we drove there, I sat in the backseat, overwhelmed with anticipation. My family played singing games in the car on the way there, but all I could think about was that crispy crust and spicy-sweet sauce. My dad ordered the famous Sicilian pie, which consisted of ten large, thick squares. Before we even got home, we would polish off a pizza in the car. He got four pieces, my sister and my mother split three slices between them, and the rest was all for me. I could do it, too—three huge, thick square chunks of pizza for the ravenous child. My mom said I ate like a truck driver. My dad called it "a healthy appetite." It was just part of our family: "Jennifer loves her food." That's what he always said, and it was true.

But I never felt full. Even when we drove to Coney Island, where my father ordered five hot dogs (two for him, one for each of us) and three orders of fries (two for him, one for the rest of us to split), it was never enough. Inevitably, I begged for another hot dog with sauerkraut and mustard, and if that wasn't enough, then I pleaded for not one but two Carvel Flying Saucers—the best ice cream cookie sandwiches I knew.

In those good old days, my family lived in a tiny house in Brooklyn. Every morning, my father went off to work. Every evening, he came home for dinner with a pocket full of candy just for me. "Jennifer loves her food," he would say. My dad was a movie star to me, a handsome man with sky-blue eyes that lit up when he saw me. He was a big-time music producer. I was in awe of him. He made my sister and I laugh with silly jokes and tricks, and he introduced me to all the great old movies.

My mom was beautiful, funny, vivacious, and full of life. A former model, she was always busy trying something new, but her passion was decorating. She was perpetually working on improving some aspect of our home, or of someone else's home, and she had a special gift for flower arranging. Everybody loved my mother. She brought energy and spirit to the room.

I idolized my big sister, of course, who was as cool as anyone could be. I lived for those days when she hung out with me. We made up dance routines together, and when I was scared at night, she let me crawl into her small single bed and scrunch up close to her so I could fall asleep.

Brooklyn was my childhood heaven. My sister and I played outside with the other kids on our block, or sat on the front stoop and watched the world go by, but more than anything, Brooklyn was about two things: community and food. The neighborhood was always out and about, doing things together. If anyone had a backyard barbeque, everyone was invited. We loved our block parties, when everyone brought out their special recipes and the treats went on for miles. But my favorite was the Italian street festival at the end of our block, held every August. My sister and I would go out together— the one place in public she would always agree to take me, her baby sister—to buy zeppolis. Zeppolis were my favorite street fair food—

perfect, hot bits of fried dough luxuriously coated in powdered sugar. As soon as we stepped out our front door, we smelled them, the aroma wafting down the street. Those fried balls of dough were love in a paper bag—love that left grease smears on our cheeks and clouds of powdered sugar in the air. What could be more luscious than eating warm zeppolis with the grease soaking spots in their brown paper holders while strolling through the Brooklyn streets with my big sister? Nothing in my life was more perfect than that.

But although my life felt good and right, and I loved Brooklyn and my family, I struggled with health issues throughout my childhood. I had chronic, severe ear infections requiring course after course of antibiotics, and I ran mysterious high fevers that required emergency room visits and ice baths. My mother had to hold me in the ice water bath while I screamed and shivered. She cried while she held me down, but my fever was 104 degrees and the doctor said she had to do it to keep me from having a seizure. Then I would be okay again, for a while. Sometimes, my stomach hurt. Sometimes, I felt nervous, for no apparent reason. Then a fever would come on again. But what did all of that matter, when I had food to comfort me, and a family I adored, and a community that kept me safe and secure?

WHEN MY MOTHER was diagnosed with stage 3 cervical cancer, life began to change. It's the first bad thing that I ever remember happening to our family. I was far too young to understand what was really going on. Cancer was a strange and foreign word to me. All I really knew was that my mother wasn't well. When she was home, she stayed in her room resting, and from an early age, I knew not to bother her. When she came out, we all spoke in soft voices. Sometimes, she picked me up and cradled me in her arms. She was weak and her knees gave out when she walked, but she told me later that she used to hold me when she had to walk because she knew that if she was holding me, she wouldn't let herself fall. Often, she wasn't home at all, but in the hospital for treatments, and because my father was usually at work and my sister was at school, I was left with a babysitter most of the time. The babysitter was a heavy woman who plopped me in front of the TV every day with a big plate of food. I ate and watched TV all day, waiting for my father and my sister to come home.

At least I had food and entertainment. I was enraptured by the movies and TV shows featuring beautiful actresses. I wanted to be one of them. It was a fantasy world that was magical and amazing from my young perspective. Those hours in front of the television were an education, and they demonstrated to my young mind something I could aspire to—something that could help people forget their troubles, because that's what television did for me.

Every now and then, when the babysitter wasn't available, I went to the hospital with my mother, where I quickly learned that I had the power to cheer everyone up. I performed the dance routines I'd invented with my sister while I waited for my mother's treatment to be over. All the nurses came to watch and bring me candy. Sometimes, my mom was there, too. The way she looked so happy to see me dance and carry on in front of everyone was better than applause. Her favorite was my Cher routine. I put a jacket on my head and swayed back and forth, each long sleeve swinging like her long hair as I sang, "Babe…I got you, babe!" Everyone laughed and clapped and smiled. The attention was great, but even more, I felt so happy in that moment, recognizing that I was making other people happy. It's probably one of the reasons I became an actress.

When my mother was back home, we all looked forward to the nights when she felt well enough to come downstairs for dinner. After she got sick, there were so few times when we were all together that those dinners—the whole family, plus food!—were filled with meaning and contentment. When food was on the table, everybody seemed to get along, at least for a little while.

After my mother came home in full remission, she had constant stomach issues, even more than I remembered her having before—bloating, constipation, diarrhea. The doctors told her that the cancer had caused a hormonal imbalance, and they blamed all her symptoms on it. So did she. She always said she had a "sensitive stomach...because of the hormones." To this day, that's what she says: "It's because of the hormones."

But it wasn't just her stomach, it also seemed to be her nerves. I don't know exactly when the panic attacks started, but when they happened, I could see it coming. My usually outgoing, funny, and talkative mother would get very quiet. Then she would begin to blink her eyes a lot. Then she would start to sweat, and then it would be time to leave. She had to get out of wherever we were at the time, as quickly as possible. It was always an emergency. "I have to get out of here," she whispered, and then I knew whatever fun we were having was over. It didn't matter where we were or what was happening. Her attacks meant I was pulled out of stores, away from birthday parties, or sometimes we just turned the car around and went back home, never even getting to where we were going. She fled to her bedroom, closed the door, and stayed in there for hours.

My mother was always a mystery to me. She was committed to doing things—getting out, traveling, seeing the world, having experiences, like taking the family to Disney World for Christmas, or to the Bahamas on vacation, or a bus trip through the Rocky Mountains with my sister and my grandmother. Sometimes, we vacationed with my cousins, at a place called Pleasant Acres in the Catskills. A remote little old-style resort, Pleasant Acres had shuffleboard and ping pong, but the best part was the cafeteria. A bell rang, as if summoning cattle, three times a day. Shockingly, I was always the first to arrive. Whatever they served, I piled it on my plate and ate it all. "Jennifer loves her food," my father would say—that old refrain.

But despite her fervent desire to get out into the world, at the same time, my mother was always fearful that her health issues would get in the way. It wasn't just her stomach, it was the anxiety. On that bus trip, as the bus wound along a narrow mountain road, my mother freaked out and had to get off. She tried to pay someone to drive her back down so she could wait for everyone else at the bottom. The bus driver spent thirty minutes trying to convince her that the bus would be a safer ride down.

As I grew older, her attacks grew longer. Sometimes, she stayed in her room for days at a time. Finally, our family stopped traveling because my mother was too afraid to get on an airplane. If we went anywhere, we would drive, and whether or not we would actually make it all the way to our destination was always a great big question mark. We began to miss more family functions as my mother withdrew. Mostly, I missed my father's family: his brother and sister-in-law, and their two children, Genine, who was my age, and Phillip, who was a couple of years younger. Genine loved food almost as much as I did, and her house was amazing to me—it had a half-underground pool and big rooms, and, compared to our tiny home in Brooklyn, it seemed like a mansion to me. I loved the huge kitchen best of all. It was always stocked with tons of food. Amazing food. Food I'd only seen on television, that my mother would have never allowed into our house. All kinds of cookies, including those Oreos my father and I used to sneak on the way home from the deli. Every kind of ice cream. Boxes and boxes of candy and bright sugary cereal. And the leftovers! Breaded chicken cutlets, pasta, meatballs, a constant supply of cold cuts and cheese. Our family's special 'weekend foods' were available 24/7 at Genine's house. It was a perpetual and extravagant feast.

When we got together with my cousins for the holidays, whatever emotional traumas or resentments or issues were brewing within or between our respective families were ceremoniously swept away as soon as the food arrived. Holidays exceeded my wildest dreams: Christmas dinner started with my grandmother's homemade manicotti covered in sauce. Then clams, more pasta, fish salad, cookies from the local bakery, ice cream, cream puffs, pastry, and my Aunt Roe's famous carrot cake, a delight I thought about all year.

Oh, that carrot cake. There was just something about it. It represented a higher echelon of gastronomic achievement to me. Most of my childhood sugar cravings centered around chocolate—Oreos, chocolate donuts, rainbow cookies, chocolate peanut butter cups. That carrot cake was something from another realm—ethereal, light. It was an *adult cake*. A happy cake, with the magic power to imbue those who ate it with serenity, with this sense of joy and contentment. All without chocolate! That was amazing to me, as a child.

Bringing out the cake was always an event, and my aunt would make the most of it. She knew exactly how everyone felt about that mystical, transcendent cake. I could barely contain myself: two layers of spicy, sweet, tender goodness flecked with *carrots,* of all things, but who would ever know it, with those layers of delectable, decadent cream cheese frosting and the ring of crunchy walnuts around the top?

But as my mother's behavior became more and more unpredictable because of her health and because of other brewing hostilities among our families, we began to cancel. This caused a lot of tension within the family. Relatives called her flighty and flaky, among other things. I felt for my mother because I knew her health wasn't her fault, and the mean things family members were saying weren't fair. At the same time, I still wanted her to be "normal." When people began to call her "Crazy Phyllis," my mother pretended to be amused by it, but I hated it. Nobody knew better than my sister and I what it was like to live with her unpredictable health and moods. Every Christmas, my sister and I, all dressed up for dinner at my grandmother's house, sat together on the landing of the stairs, waiting as quietly as possible, listening to my mother say we were not going, and my father say we were going, back and forth. Sometimes, we waited for hours for the final decision. My sister put her arm around me, knowing I was so very sad at the prospect of not getting to go.

This kind of arguing back and forth soon became a weekend event, no longer exclusive to the holidays. Whatever the fight was about, it usually culminated in my mother proclaiming, "I'm leaving!" I dreaded those words. I loved my mom and I wanted her to stay. What would happen to the family without her? But she never actually left. Her up-and-down, back-and-forth behavior was something I didn't understand, and it scared me. At least on those much-anticipated Christmas outings, my mother almost always gave in, and we eventually got to my grandmother's house. Tensions were high, nobody speaking on the car ride over. I knew an abrupt departure was inevitable. Burying my face and fears in the food when I arrived calmed the world around me for the moment, and extended into slow motion those brief lovely hours I clung to, when the whole family sat together, laughing and eating and celebrating.

Sometimes, I believed my mother enjoyed the name "Crazy Phyllis" and made the most of it. I knew that personally, she suffered, but as a child, I always wondered whether it would be an up day or a down day. Would she dote on me or would I lose her for a week or more? She might be the life of the party, or she might fly into a rage, or she might just disappear into her bedroom. Sometimes, her anger was entirely justified. My father wasn't an easy man to live with by any stretch of the imagination, and she endured many disappointments in her life, as well as extended family judgments. At other times, however, her anger seemed to come from nowhere. We never knew what might trigger it. Often on edge, walking on eggshells. I never wanted to flip her switch. Along with the anger, came severe stomach issues and a recurrence of her panic attacks.

I spent much of my childhood fearful, anxious, and overwhelmed by a deep sadness I couldn't define, but that was always there, simmering underneath everything I did, even when I was running around with my cousins, playing and laughing. I became quiet and withdrawn, or boisterous and seeking attention, which made people whisper about me—was I inheriting her "moods"? One moment I was carousing with my cousins or putting on a show in the living room, and then, the next moment, I faded away into myself. People began to call me "her mother's daughter," and while that scared me, it was what it was. My mother was awesome when she was feeling well, and I loved her madly. I was proud to be her daughter. She was dealing with her life and her health in the best way she knew how. I would do the same.

It wasn't a perfect family. My father was often away, consumed by his career and constantly worried about money. My sister was quickly becoming a typical teenager who no longer wanted her baby sister following her around all the time. My mother, well…we never knew what was in store with her. But it was family—it was loud and raucous and wonderful, and it was mine. Then we moved to Staten Island, and everything changed again.

MY SISTER WAS crying to my mom in the kitchen one afternoon and I ran in to see what had happened. Her eyes were swollen with tears. She had just started high school and was refusing to go over the bridge to live in the "sticks," as she called it. Being my sister's shadow, I agreed, complaining loudly that I wouldn't be caught dead in "the sticks" either, even though I had no idea what she meant. I had always thought of Staten Island as "the country" because, from my eight-year-old urban perspective, that's what it was: large wide streets and big houses with lawns that took up half the sidewalk. Huge trees and underground pools. Staten Island was the place we went on holidays to visit my father's brother, and, most importantly, that was where my cousin Genine lived, in her magnificent house. To me, Staten Island was a beautiful, mysterious, wealthy place. A place full of food.

So, when I heard we were moving to Staten Island, and then, when I found out we were moving into *my cousin's exact house* because my uncle was buying a bigger house in affluent Todt Hill, I was overwhelmed. We were moving into a mansion! I wondered if the house would come fully stocked with all that food! Had we become one of those rich families? It seemed too good to be true.

My mother explained that my Dad was rising higher and higher in his career, so this was the time, whether my sister liked it or not. That was the end of it. There would be no arguing. We moved everything out of our cute little 950-square-foot home in Brooklyn with the patch of grass out front and the little pool my dad set up and took down with the change of seasons, into Genine's house—2,500 square feet, curiously suburban, strangely quiet. We had a big manicured lawn, but we didn't have a front stoop. There was no bakery or deli at the end of the block. No sign of a street fair. Not even an inkling that we might live in a neighborhood. Just house after house after house along winding streets, with no indication of where a block might begin or end.

My parents told me it was a "better" house, but once we began to move all our things in and make it our own, I had doubts. Where was all the food? The cupboards stood empty and the house held no trace of my cousin or the fun we had. I stood in the driveway looking down the street, first one way and then another. Nobody played outside. Nobody was sitting on their stoops. They didn't even have stoops! How would I know who my automatic friends were? Where was I? The street and all its perfectly manicured lawns and beautiful houses felt empty and dead to me. It was lovely, of course, and wealthy, but why didn't the air move? Why were the trees so still? Where were all the kids?

I quickly internalized that quiet loneliness, increasing my natural tendency towards melancholy that came from somewhere I didn't really understand. I spent a lot of time in my room, listening to music and writing poetry and feeling lonely and sad.

Starting third grade in a new school didn't make things any better. Everyone was already established in their cliques and I was an outsider. Making friends wasn't easy for me. It didn't help that my sister told me that Brooklyn was cool and Staten Island definitely was not. I believed her, so I had a slight chip on my shoulder. What I knew for sure was that it didn't feel like a community in the way Brooklyn had. I thought I would see my cousin Genine more often, but I didn't. She went to a different school.

I was growing into my awkward stage at this time in my life. My teeth sported huge gaps when my baby teeth fell out and my eye-teeth didn't appear on schedule. We waited and waited for the new teeth but they were no-shows, so my other teeth spread out, leaving me feeling freakish and uneven. The dentist said he supposed I was born without those teeth. Nobody thought much about it. Finally, to my delight, one began to grow in—a spindly, twisted tooth which quickly chipped and then fell out soon after. "It's just the way she was born," the doctor told my mother. These were the days when polite and responsible adults never questioned a medical doctor, so my mom just accepted this non-diagnosis and told me that the gaps in my smile gave me character. I tried to believe her, but I also learned to smile with my mouth closed. My mother didn't care for braces and my dad said we didn't have the money, so I ended up with a lot of character, and all the teasing that goes with that.

WHEN MY FATHER lost his job, our family life began to unravel. He struggled to find another job that was as good as the one he had lost, but in the meantime, in order to pay the bills, he worked under his younger brother on Wall Street. It was meant to be a temporary position. Little did we know he would keep that job for the rest of his working days. Working on Wall Street wasn't his passion, and from the moment my father left the music business, the sparkle left his eyes. He became an invisible member of the household as the years wore on. He was physically there, but that was all. I clung to the memories of our times together in Brooklyn and tried to think of him that way, even though that part of him seemed far away, a distant memory. My mother's moods continued to be uneven, but she was determined to do something more with her life. She loved to decorate our house, and she was good at it, so she made a small business out of it. She started taking decorating jobs here and there, so she was out of the house more frequently. When I came home from school, more often than not, I was alone.

One family highlight of the year was Christmas, when my father took the three of us into the city to marvel at the big Christmas tree in Rockefeller Center. We always drove by it—we never actually got out of the car because my dad didn't want to deal with the traffic and my mom was afraid of the city—but even from the car, the energy was palpable. Extraordinary. We always had dinner at Benihana, and I loved how they cooked the food right in front of us. I practically licked that thick, savory sauce off my plate. In the evening, a holiday magic fell over the city. The lights, the towering buildings, the air that was completely unlike that static Staten Island air that I felt. It seemed like anything was possible in Manhattan. I couldn't believe such a place was just a bridge or a ferry ride away. It was a completely different world! I told myself I would live there someday. I belonged in the city. But I wasn't living in the city yet. I was still a kid, and I had a long road ahead of me. Then the stomach aches started.

The first time my stomach decided to make a fool out of me was when I threw up all over the stage during my first play in sixth grade. It was the school Christmas show, and I was picked to sing "Silent Night" in front of the entire school. When I opened my mouth to sing the first line, I vomited. As soon as it happened, I stood very still and stared out at the audience, in shock and horror and self-disgust. Then, I burst into tears and ran from the stage.

Nausea and stomach issues increased in frequency as I got older. The doctor said I had a "nervous stomach," just like my mother. I began to live in constant fear that I might not have easy access to a bathroom, or that I might humiliate myself again and throw up in the middle of some high-stakes social situation, or anywhere with an audience of any kind, especially at school. I began to adopt my mother's stomach regimen: I lived on bagels, crackers, pasta, and toast. My mother told me these foods soaked up the stomach acid, and who would know better than my mother how to handle an unpredictable stomach? She was the expert, with decades of experience.

When I hit puberty, my health issues became even more unsettling. Once my "monthly visitor" arrived, the sports I'd always played were out of the question. My symptoms were so severe and unpredictable that I couldn't risk being on a team that depended on me. The bloating and swelling were so uncomfortable that I could barely move, let alone compete. As I drifted away from sports, I lost my last real connection with my father. He never missed my games and it was the one thing we still did together. Now, that was gone, too.

Then the depression began. I'd had a melancholy feeling ever since I could remember, but this was stronger. I was (and still am) extremely sensitive to the world around me. I thought deeply about things, but now I seemed to be on overdrive. The doctor said it was my hormones, but that didn't make sense to me because my dark moods lasted all month long. I couldn't snap out of it. I tried to cheer myself up, but I was in a dark hole and I couldn't climb out.

Meanwhile, my sister was gone a lot, often out with her boyfriends or her friends, but she also had extreme bouts of illness, like strep throat and then extreme fatigue. She was diagnosed with anemia and she was almost always on antibiotics for something. Then, my grandmother, my mother's mother, had to move in with us.

My grandmother, Bernadette, and I were very close, and we got even closer when she moved into our home. She was a tiny woman of just eighty pounds, increasingly frail but always elegant and dignified. She used to sit with me and tell me that I could be an actress, that I could be anything. She also suffered from the family "nervous stomach," and her pain and bathroom issues were humiliating to her. She was trapped by her nervous stomach, much like my mother was, and I could see that she hoped for something more for me. It broke my heart to see how she struggled. She tried to hide it by dressing up immaculately every day and sitting primly on the couch like a proper lady should, but I heard her moaning in pain in her room at night, behind the closed door. When she was finally forced to have a colostomy bag, she was devastated. She couldn't keep food down or weight on herself, and the doctors never knew why. We could all see she didn't have long to live, and it was tragic for us to watch her dwindle in such an undignified and heartbreaking way. She was seventy-eight years old when she died of cancer. I took her name as my middle name at my confirmation.

After my grandmother was gone, my mother's attacks continued to get worse. Each time, she disappeared into her bedroom with a bowl of cereal as her only nourishment. Sometimes, I peeked into the room and saw her staring, catatonic, at the television. Sometimes, I snuck in quietly and asked if I could lie with her. When she nodded, I crawled into bed, being careful not to be too rough, so I wouldn't disturb her, and rested my head on her hip.

This was the beginning of a strange bonding ritual with my mother. When I started high school, I was the only one she let into her world. Sometimes, she asked me if I wanted to stay home from school and hang out with her. Of course, my answer was yes. I loved these times, even though they revolved around some sort of mutual sadness. We shared our depression and even reveled in it. Instead of driving me to school, my mother drove through McDonalds (both of us still in our pajamas) and picked up Egg McMuffins, pancakes, and apple pies, then took them home and ate them in bed while watching *Donahue*. My mother talked to me a lot about her life, fears, and frustrations. She shared things a mother probably shouldn't burden her child with, but she had to talk to someone and I was the one who was there to listen and understand. She talked about my father a lot, and she also talked about her health, and how I had inherited her issues. She hated that she had passed this burden on to me. I suspected that if it weren't for her health issues, she would be living a very different life. I think that's why she always encouraged me to go out and change my fate. She wanted for me what she'd been unable to achieve for herself. Part of me was honored and flattered that I was the one allowed into her world, that I was the one she told things to that probably nobody else knew. Another part of me wondered if I was seeing my future in her. But she needed me, and I liked that.

My school wasn't quite so impressed with my attendance record. One day, they called to report that I had been gone twenty-two days in one year, and even one more day would result in my being held back. My mother was surprised, as if she hadn't even considered that taking me out of school was a problem. It's not that school wasn't important to her, but being smart in school wasn't really on her radar. She was smart in other ways. At this point, even without a high school diploma, she had managed to become an award-winning decorator known around Staten Island for her skill. She wanted even more for me. That's when I realized how important it was for me to get out of Staten Island. It couldn't just be a dream for me. I had to make it happen.

I already had a plan, first hatched in those early days watching television when my mother was in the hospital. When I first told my parents I wanted to be an actress, my father's first response was, "The most important thing a woman can do is to get her stenography and typing skills down, so she can always get a job if she has to."

"Fuck that," my mother replied, not surprising me. "You go for the world," she said, pointing at me accusingly, as if I had considered doing anything less. "Never depend on anyone but yourself. Never depend on a man for anything!" The dig at my father wasn't lost on me.

I've never forgotten those words. It probably wasn't the best advice for blissful future relationships, but it has made me strong and self-reliant. My mother was the one who dropped me off in front of a movie theater when I was thirteen years old and told me to go in and get a job. I became the candy girl (I ate enough popcorn to last me a lifetime), and I haven't stopped working since. But ever since those early days, I had my dream in mind. I wanted to be like those women I saw on the screen at the movie theater. They were strong. They were independent. They had real careers, and they made a very impressionable young girl happy when she watched them. I wanted to do the same. I wanted it all.

So many girls I knew dreamed of marrying their high school sweethearts, having babies, and never leaving the neighborhood. That's all wonderful if that's what you choose, but it wasn't what I wanted. I knew even as a child that I wanted to explore the world, be independent, be fearless, and taste everything life had to serve up. Stomach pains or no stomach pains, I had to do it—for my grandmother, for my mother, for myself.

3

triggers

In eighth grade, we had an assignment. We were all asked to write what we wanted to be when we grew up. It never occurred to me to hold back. I had a plan, and I was simply answering the question. I was going to be an actress!

That was a mistake. They published my dream in the school yearbook, and I became an object of ridicule. Everyone made fun of me. The girls followed me around, taunting me: "You think who you are?" they jeered, which was their version of, "Who do you think you are?" They yelled at me from down the hall or down the street, "You think you're so great, you think you can be an actress?"

"Why do you think *you* can be an actress!"

"Yeah, you *think* who you are!"

I didn't understand it. Didn't anyone else have big dreams? I felt like everybody else already knew which way their lives would go, almost as if the decisions were already laid out for them and they liked it that way. Since I wasn't following the same protocol, that laid me open to ridicule. I quickly learned not to share any more dreams. In high school, I never participated in anything remotely resembling acting, for fear of ridicule. Around this time, peer pressure became an even greater source of stress than my home life. Most of my friends went to a different school, so I was a loner. I lived in an Italian-Catholic neighborhood, where some of the biggest mafia families lived. "Mafia" meant nothing to me beyond what I'd seen in the *Godfather* movies, but what I did know is that some of the kids in my neighborhood were tough. Really tough. And they seemed extremely angry. The violence I saw in my neighborhood coming from these young people was like something you would see in the very best mob film. It was no joke. They all showed up to church on Sunday, then beat the hell out of each other the rest of the week. The hypocrisy shocked me and I wanted no part of it.

In my first year of Catholic high school, I dated a very rough boy from this group. He was my first boyfriend, and, in retrospect, I realize just how abusive the relationship was, although, at the time, it seemed normal, like every other relationship I saw. People around me, adults included, communicated by screaming, throwing things, and calling each other awful names. Because it was so much a part of the culture, I didn't see anything unusual about it. I thought this was just how people acted.

The boyfriend was scary, but eventually I got away from him. He was nothing compared to the mob girls. They were more like caged animals than girls, and who could blame them? Now that I'm older, I know what it means to be from a mafia family, and I can only imagine how difficult it was for them. They were angry in a truly violent way I'd never seen in women or girls before. They lashed out at anyone they could find who seemed different than they were—and that was me.

Those girls tortured me. Maybe a boy they liked looked my way, or a friend of a friend said God-knows-what about me, but whatever it was, I felt like they genuinely wanted to kill me—and they told me they did, many times over. Whenever I saw this gang of girls, I trembled from inside, like my stomach was vibrating.

I had seen my mother have anxiety attacks, but I never understood how it felt on a personal level until I was fifteen years old. My parents were dropping me off at a school dance, and I knew some of the mob girls would be there. My very small group of friends was already there, but I feared they wouldn't be able to protect me. As my parents drove me to the dance, I began to get more nervous. When we pulled up to the school, a wave of fear came over me that was so intense, I refused to get out of the car. I'd had unexplained waves of nervousness before, but nothing like this. My stomach felt like it was going to explode, and my heart raced with such a fury that I felt as though I might be having a heart attack. I couldn't go in. I couldn't even move.

"I can't do it," I said. "I can't go in."

My mother turned around and looked at me. "What's wrong?"

I told her that my chest felt tight, my stomach felt sick, and I couldn't breathe. In a moment, she knew exactly what was going on.

"I know what this is," she said. "You're having an anxiety attack." She said it as if it was a normal, coming-of-age experience for everyone. "Don't let this stop you," she said, firmly, looking me in the eyes. "You have to overcome it. You have to go in."

It seemed impossible. I started to hyperventilate. "Breathe," she told me, trying to calm me down, but it was to no avail. That was when she reached into her bag of tricks and gave me my first Valium. "Here. Take this. It will calm you down." She hated seeing me go through such terrible anxiety, and this was the way she knew how to cope. She tried her best to talk me into going and having fun and not letting it get to me, but it was hopeless. I couldn't go. I felt sick to my stomach. We drove home in silence.

This was my first anxiety attack. Was it from the fear of getting jumped, or was it something else? I didn't know at the time, but the attacks continued, even when I wasn't faced with a prospect as terrifying as bullies. Every anxiety attack brought with it the feeling that my stomach would explode, and vice versa—it seemed like whenever my stomach hurt, anxiety would soon follow. My depression also came more frequently, along with bursts of anger and constant exhaustion. My doctors continued to explain it away by blaming hormones, or "just being a teenager," but deep inside, I knew something wasn't right.

Finally, when my stomach problems became debilitating, my mother took me to the doctor yet again, and they agreed to give me a barium enema, to see if they could find anything wrong. It was a humiliating experience for a teenage girl. I had to hold a ton of liquid in my bladder while being poked and prodded and having my stomach X-rayed. All the while, the doctor performing the test seemed angry. Finally, she turned to me.

"Why are you having this test? There's obviously nothing wrong with you."

I stared at her. She was the doctor. Didn't she know? "Because… something's wrong with my stomach?" I ventured.

She rolled her eyes. "You mean you're pregnant?"

"No!" I was shocked—I was still a virgin! Why didn't she believe I was really sick? How could she go *there?* But, sure enough, the results of the test were negative. It was the first time I was officially disregarded by doctors, who concluded there really was nothing wrong with me. It must be in my head. (At least, they had to admit I wasn't pregnant.) It was also the first time I saw that look—the look doctors give people when they think the symptoms are made up. The look that labels you a hypochondriac. It was also the first time I wondered if all my stomach pain might actually be in my head. Was this all in my imagination? Deep down, I knew it was physical. It *felt* physical. But the look in that doctor's eyes made me doubt myself. I was a teenager and the person doubting me was not just an adult but a doctor. I couldn't help feeling like I was wasting everybody's time even being there in the office, and I should just quit all this nonsense-talk at once. That my pain shouldn't be anyone else's problem.

Meanwhile, my mom was trying to help me in the best way she could. She hated seeing me like this. She told me not to let those girls, or my anxiety, or my stomach issues, or my extreme depression get to me. She said, and these were her exact words: "The next time you feel that anger that comes out of you, you go and punch one of those girls in the face when she comes near you. You'll feel better!" I wanted to tell her it wasn't so easy, but, then again, I knew that she knew exactly how difficult it was to feel so unwell so much of the time, while also battling anxiety that wouldn't let up.

The next wave of symptoms came when my fatigue became debilitating. This wasn't just my usual exhaustion. This was an *I cannot move my limbs* sort of exhaustion. When my mother took me back to the doctor, this time I got a diagnosis: mononucleosis. (I would later learn that a virus in childhood can trigger an autoimmune disease—was this the one? Or was it one of those fevers I had as a young child?) It was so severe a case, I was hospitalized for four days with a raging fever. When I got sick, I got *sick*. My illnesses were always extreme. Just like the ear infections from my infancy, I took mono to the nth degree. The doctor said the mono took over because my immune system was so weak. I missed weeks of school and took weeks of antibiotics.

Even after I was supposedly recovered, my sleeping patterns were outrageous. I had a terrible time getting out of bed in the morning. I dragged through school and couldn't wait to come home to sleep. Every afternoon, I arrived home to an empty house. My mother was usually off doing some decorating project or teaching a flower-arranging class or doing the flowers for somebody's wedding. She was also working as a decorator out of a local carpet store, trying her best to make something of her own life. My sister and father were out working, too. I dragged myself into the kitchen and stood in front of an empty refrigerator—my mother hated to food-shop—with a ravenous appetite only slightly stronger than my exhaustion. Most days, I either ordered a pizza or made pasta with peas and butter and ate every bite, then collapsed on my bed and slept for hours. When everyone got home, I ate dinner, barely made it through my shift at the movie theater, then went right back to sleep until the last possible minute before school. This became the routine of my adolescence.

At one point, my exhaustion was so severe that I began to lose muscle movement in my face. Everything drooped and my legs felt like silly putty. I knew something was very wrong, but I stalled on going to the doctor. I was tired of being humiliated and reprimanded. When it lasted for several months, my mother finally insisted. We went back to the doctor to demand answers. He said I had some sort of facial palsy. He took some blood and a few days later, he said I had the Epstein-Barr virus. The doctor blamed it on my severe mono and said the virus would never leave my body. Great. Just great.

Extreme exhaustion and weakness became my constant companions. The doctor said there was no remedy. When the dropping face muscles started to tingle, the doctor sent me for an MRI to check for multiple sclerosis. The results were negative again. I didn't have MS. They sent me home with my first prescription to visit a therapist. My mom said that was ridiculous. I didn't need a therapist. I just needed my own bag of tricks. Valium and saltines and Pepto-Bismol. And we pushed on.

Then my mom got the idea that some real exercise would help me. I agreed, but only out of vanity. I was getting thicker. I had been a gymnast as a child so I had always been muscular, but lately I just felt bloated and large. I blamed my long hours of sleeping and intensive carb binges. My body was becoming very uncomfortable. Maybe exercise *would* help. I joined a local gym.

WORKING OUT DID make me feel a little bit better, and I loved it. Within a few months, I was working there. I taught aerobics and sculpting classes, but I was most fascinated by the people who were weight training. Before I knew it, they were letting me teach a weight training class! (How anyone ever allowed me to do this without any formal training is beyond me!) I was a dedicated worker and took my job and my fitness seriously, and I learned a lot from the older teachers. My classes became very popular and I got stronger. I was still exhausted, but I had less time at home to binge on pizza and pasta. All they had lying around the gym was fruit, so I noshed on that all the time. I was feeling better—but the stress was still ever-present. I was still being chased and harassed by the mob girls, and one afternoon at work, they came for me.

I don't know what I'd done this time, in their minds. They waited for me to get off work, and as soon as I came out of the gym, they surrounded me. I was petrified. But even more than that, I was done with being petrified. One girl took her drink and poured it over my head, then threw the cup in my face and cursed and screamed at me that I was a whore. (I was still a virgin at this point.) Then she said she was going to kill me, and she went for me.

Slightly in shock but so absolutely over being tormented, I blocked her swings and started screaming back. I think these girls were as surprised as I was. Some adults from the gym I worked at started to walk over. The girls turned around and walked back to their pimped out cars. As they drove off, they yelled out the car windows that they would have me and my family killed, and that fat dog that sat on my lawn, too.

I don't know exactly what changed in me that day, but I realized then, more than ever before, that I didn't have to accept the life that I was living and the circumstances I'd been given. I did keep my dog inside after that (just in case), but I felt more inspired than ever to go out and create the life that I wanted. I had a few more months to go before I finished high school, so I decided I had to start laying the groundwork. I had to have a plan.

I BEGAN TO visit the city on my own every chance I could get. By the time I was seventeen years old, I knew the city pretty well, and all it had to offer. I wanted every drop of it for myself. My parents set my curfew at a ridiculous 10 p.m., but when I wanted to go out and venture into the city, I told them I was sleeping at a friend's house. Then my friends and I drove to Manhattan and danced all night in clubs. It was pure freedom.

I plowed through my fatigue and caught up on my sleep whenever I could. In the city, I felt completely at home. My friends and I made it a point of pride to get into the clubs where they only let in the "beautiful people." As cute teenage girls with fake IDs, we usually got sent straight to the front of the line. Life was looking up—I couldn't wait to make it permanent.

One night, as I was dancing my butt off at a club called Mars that was notoriously hard to get into, a couple approached me.

"Excuse me," the woman said. "Are you a dancer?"

I was flattered, and I laughed. "No."

"Have you ever watched MTV?" the man said.

My father would never pay for cable TV in a million years, but I lied. "MTV? Of course! I love MTV!"

They looked at each other, and the woman smiled. "How would you like to come dance for Club MTV, hosted by Downtown Julie Brown? We think you'd be great."

I nearly wet myself.

Remaining cool and a bit hesitant—my parents had told me all the stories about young girls who go to the big city and never come back—I gave them my number. They gave me an address and a time to show up. They also said to bring many changes of clothes because they would be taping a bunch of shows at once.

I was beside myself. Club MTV! Downtown Julie Brown! Even without cable TV, I knew exactly what this meant. A week later, I was nervous beyond belief. I packed a bag of the coolest clothes I had and headed to the city in my old, beat-up red Honda, blasting Mary J. Blige and singing loudly to distract myself from my flip-flopping stomach. Part of me was scared that I was going to be kidnapped and sold into a life of porn, but I kept hearing my mother's voice: "You can do anything you really want to do." I would be brave! Despite my reservations and my crazy health, I knocked on a small, black, ominous backstage door. When it opened, as scared as I was, I felt right at home. The room was full of young people, all different and all full of life, dancing around and talking. The energy in the room was enough to make me forget any of my ills, at least for the moment. Because there I was on the set of Club MTV, and, just like that, I became a Club MTV dancer.

Soon, I became one of their featured dancers, along with a girl named Camille. She was older and had been there long before me, so she already knew how it all worked. I befriended her and she showed me the ins and outs of being on the show. Along with some others, we were both hired out to show up at private parties and even bat mitzvahs as the MTV dancers. Crazy as it seems, I felt like I was living the dream. It's funny to me now, but I was just so happy to be around these other goal-oriented people who all had dreams and all spoke about them freely. It felt like I was a million miles away from home.

I still suffered with health issues. When the parties we were hired to do were a few hours outside the city, I got tremendous anxiety. My stomach was always an issue, but then I would hear my mother's voice: "Don't let it stop you!" I was never without my bag of tricks—the crackers, the Pepto Bismol, a bottle of ginger ale. One day, my stomach hurt so much after a party that I had to make the driver pull over, in search of a bathroom. I was in a van with a bunch of kids between seventeen and nineteen years old, and there I was, begging for a bathroom stop. Humiliating! I stumbled into the restaurant bathroom and drank half the bottle of Pepto-Bismol so I could make it home without asking to stop again.

I finally graduated from high school and continued with my plan. If I wanted to be an actress, I was going to have to learn how to act. My time on MTV had given me confidence performing in front of people, so I got up the guts to take acting classes at nearby Wagner College that had just started that year. It was a start, but I was still living in Staten Island and the people around me were still fighting and yelling and hanging out in the same places and doing the same things. Something had to change.

Then, one day, I saw my escape route. After filming Club MTV, Downtown Julie Brown made an announcement that her friend's restaurant, The Coffee Shop, was hiring. The Coffee Shop was a cooler-than-cool place where all the famous people went. It was extremely hard to get in, let alone get a job there, but what an opportunity! What if I could get one of those jobs? I could meet people, I could make money—I could move out! I had already saved about $1,000 from working and from a small inheritance I got when my grandmother passed away. I knew if I could get a job, that would be enough to get me set up until my first paycheck. I had to try.

I arrived at The Coffee Shop to find that a lot of other people had the same idea. The line was huge. Then they began to divide us into two lines. Soon, I realized that one line was full of people who "looked the part," and the other line was full of people who didn't. I bristled a little at this blatant prejudice. Were looks all that mattered? What about work ethic? What about responsibility? But I was in the line of "desirables," and I was hired that day. I kept my complaints to myself. This was no time to take a stand. This was a time to grab the opportunity.

I started immediately. I worked the graveyard shift with a group of other young hopefuls, all of us with desire, passion, and big dreams. I wanted to fill up every moment with these new, inspiring friends, and push all the old obstacles out of my old life forever. We waited tables until the wee hours of the morning, and then we would go out dancing until the sun came up. The exhaustion was tough but the sheer exhilaration of freedom kept me going. Within a month, I had saved another couple of hundred dollars. I enrolled in the famous Lee Strasberg Institute for Acting, got an apartment in a terrible neighborhood with one of my co-workers, and moved out of my parent's home a few weeks before my nineteenth birthday.

A new chapter in my life had begun, and I was psyched beyond words. I vowed that I would never let anything or anyone stop me from going in the direction I was headed. Unfortunately, there were roadblocks ahead that were determined to stop me.

4

living the dream

My apartment was cramped and the neighborhood was dodgy, and my roommate, another wannabe actress named Natalie, was everything I was not. She was petite and dainty with a small-boned frame and rich long black hair, and she ate like a bird. I had bleached my hair like Madonna, and I was tall (next to her), and I felt huge whenever I was around her, especially when she told me that I should pay more in rent because I ate way more than she did, and took up most of the refrigerator space. But my life was completely different than it had been before, and it was all completely fine with me.

I was free, and freedom from my past also meant I could buy and eat whatever I wanted. No oatmeal for me—I stocked up on everything I never got at home. Boxes of sweetened cereal, bagels every day, cream cheese and cold cuts and cookies and candy. And working at a restaurant? Forget it—that was heaven. I ate there with glee. Banana cream pie, creamed spinach, mashed potatoes. I still battled fatigue, but my new life was so exciting and I had so much hope for the future that I barreled through it. "Don't let it stop you." My mother's voice was always with me.

Soon, I was promoted to the day shift, and then I understood what all The Coffee Shop fuss was about. I waited on celebrities all the time—Lauren Hutton, Christopher Reeve, all the supermodels of the day. I heard Madonna was even in there one time when I was off. I couldn't believe I missed her! People often mistook me for her, or asked me if I was related to her. With my dye job and fashion choices, we did resemble each other—both Italian, both with those "character" spaces in our teeth, both with the same haircut.

One afternoon, a young guy sitting at the prestigious Table 7, where we were instructed to seat anybody that was anybody, stopped me as I flew by with an armful of plates.

"Excuse me," he said. "Are you related to Madonna?"

I laughed. "No, but thanks!" I turned to go—we were busy—but he stopped me again.

"Wait," he said. "Are you an actress?"

Hmm. How to answer that loaded question in New York City, where every waitress, bartender, and shop clerk had aspirations. I'd only been acting for about six months, and I wasn't making any money from it yet, but I was studying. I decided to take a leap of faith.

"I am," I said. "I'm studying at Lee Strasberg."

"You're going to be a star," he said. "I know it. Send me your headshot and I'll see if I can help you."

I nearly died. I took his info, then begged a friend to take some pictures of me so I could use them for headshots. Nothing concrete came of it—he became a well-known manager in Hollywood and today, every time I see him, we laugh about it—but, at the time, it represented something much more to me than a job. It represented possibility. My dream wasn't ridiculous. Someone out there, someone who didn't know me saw something. I would live off that hope for a long time.

This was one of the happiest times in my life. Sometimes, I worked double shifts, just to pay my rent and pay for acting school, but I loved every minute. My acting classes were the center of my world. I had one of the most difficult teachers in the school. His name was George and somehow I do believe I managed to become one of his favorites. I worked my tail off for his approval. All the students did. He was tough but no-nonsense, which I appreciated. Between work, four-hour classes, rehearsal for scene work for school, and my social life, which involved going out dancing all night after work with all my equally charged friends from the Coffee Shop, anyone would have been exhausted, but my exhaustion was extreme. My stomach woes were still prevalent, but I had my bag of tricks. I took Pepto Bismol as part of my daily routine. I would often go home just to sleep for the entire weekend. And do my laundry, of course.

By this time, I'd met my first big-city boyfriend, and that was a revelation, too. He was completely different from anyone I had ever known before. He was an artist, and he didn't yell or scream or try to beat people up. Every day, I woke up in wonderment that I had escaped what had seemed to be my fate. I was living my own life, in a world I had chosen. It almost seemed too good to be true.

IT'S FUNNY HOW one small thing can completely derail your life. One morning, I woke up with excruciating pain in my mouth, and this one small thing unleashed a beast that had been lurking just under the surface of my life.

It was a rare morning off from both acting class and work. I called my mother to complain about the pain and the swelling that was happening in my mouth even as I was telling her about it. She told me to come home and she would take me to the dentist. I called a friend to cover my afternoon shift at work and I took the ferry to Staten Island. My mom picked me up and we went straight to a dental surgeon. The verdict: I needed three wisdom teeth pulled immediately, because they were abscessed and infected. I was scared. It sounded major, and I didn't want to do it, especially when the nurse explained the after-care protocol.

"No solid food for three days," she said.

I stared at her like she was speaking a different language. No solid food? Was that even *possible?* It sounded inhumane, at the very least. My appointment wasn't for a few hours, so my mom took me to the store and we bought Jell-O and pudding in bulk. Just knowing I had those little cups at my disposal comforted me a little. I called the Coffee Shop and was able to cover all my shifts for the next couple of days. Then I went back. It was time to face the knife.

I was nervous. I had a bad feeling about the whole thing. The nurse, who was coughing and sneezing with some kind of respiratory issue, assured me that they do this surgery every day. I would be put out, and I wouldn't feel a thing. She led me into a sterile-looking white room, put me in a big chair that looked like a spaceship, and tied a bib around my neck. I tried not to look at the tray where the instruments of torture were laid out neatly around a spit bowl. Then the surgeon walked in. He seemed to be in a hurry. He told me I would be fine, and directed the nurse to start the general anesthesia. With a prick of a needle and an IV in my arm, I was out in seconds. As I felt a wave of nausea from the anesthetic, the last thing I remember thinking was, "I'll be back to my regular life in a couple of days."

The next thing I remember, I felt like I was flying around the room, but at the same time, I felt like a hundred-pound weight was holding me down. I didn't feel any pain, but I heard the nurse's voice, as if from far away, saying something to the doctor in an urgent tone. Was she upset about something? I didn't imagine it could have anything to do with me. I barely knew where I was. Then I remember opening my eyes and seeing her through a kind of fog. She was shaking me. Her voice sounded strange. "Jennifer! Jennifer, can you hear me? Jennifer, can you hear me?!"

I could see her and hear her, but I couldn't respond. It was like I wasn't in my body at all. I was watching it happen, as if it were a movie, or happening to somebody else. I couldn't move or speak, but I felt extremely calm. Then the nurse's face reared up close to me, and then the surgeon's face, with a grim scowl—and then everything went black. Then, I was back again, after a dip of unknown duration into unconsciousness, and the nurse was helping me to sit up. I still felt like I was out of my body, as the nurse brought me into another room, an empty exam room, and let me sit there for a moment. I heard her saying something about sitting up so I wouldn't swallow blood and the gauze that was in my mouth.

Then my mother was there. Everyone looked strange, as if they all wore masks. I can't explain it, but even though I could hear and see everyone, I had no real understanding of what was going on. I watched in bafflement. Was this some kind of performance? I couldn't make sense of my situation. When my mother stood right in front of me and spoke to me, I couldn't figure out the answer to her question:

"What's wrong with you?"

"She'll come out of it soon." The nurse's voice was brusque and clipped, but I wasn't entirely sure she was actually real. "Just take her home to rest." Her voice faded in and out…or was it me who was fading?

My mother took me home and I slept for twenty-four hours. When I finally woke up, I felt strange. Yes, my mouth was throbbing. Yes, my cheeks were swollen with gauze and packing, but something else was different. *I* was different. When my mother came in to check on me, I tried to explain it to her.

"Something's wrong. I don't feel like myself."

She told me to get into her big bed and she brought me pudding. I slept for a few more days. Then, we went back to the doctor so he could check that everything was fine. My mother told him I wasn't fine. Something was wrong. I was really out of it. I was non-responsive, like I wasn't there. This wasn't her daughter. He smiled indulgently.

"She's just fine," he said. "Don't worry. It just takes some time to recover, that's all." Being from the generation that trusts everything doctors say, my mom believed him. She took me home and told me I could start eating solid food. The doctor had said so.

But I was afraid to chew. I imagined I would tear open my gums. I wanted more pudding.

"We're out of pudding," my mother said. "Let me make you a bagel."

I imagined the bagel tearing my gums apart. "I'll go buy more pudding," I said.

"Are you sure?" My mother looked worried. "Do you want me to go with you?"

"No," I said, feeling a little dizzy. "I need to get some air. The doctor said I'm fine. I've got to go back out at some point. It's just up the street."

I got into my mother's car and drove the few blocks to the store. Once I got inside, I looked around for the...wait, why was I there? Where was I? I began to feel strange. Then I broke out into a cold sweat and my heart began to race. I looked around, confused. All the colors in the supermarket hurt my eyes. And the noise—people talking, cash registers jangling, cars roaring by outside—it all sounded like someone had turned up the volume on the world and then jumbled it together and dumped it into my head. Then everything sped up, like someone had pressed fast forward on a video recording. The world was moving at lightning speed. I was terrified!

I looked around, frantically trying to figure out where I was, but that just made it worse, so I put my head down and tried not to look at anything. Suddenly, a word popped into my brain: pudding. Pudding! Staring at the squares on the linoleum, trying to keep my feet moving in a straight line, I headed towards the pudding aisle. I felt like the people, the food, the shelves themselves were glaring at me, rearing up and scowling like that dental surgeon in my anesthesia-induced haze. Would the shelves fall in on me? I looked up and felt like I was on another planet. What was I looking for again? Something… Then the intensely bright walls began to close in. I had to get out of there! I couldn't even remember why I was there, or where I was. I ran out of the store, then I sat down on the curb to catch my breath. I was drenched in sweat and trembling.

I had to get home. How did I get here? Did I come in a car? My mother's car! But what did it look like? I couldn't remember. I stood up, shaking. Maybe if I saw it, I would recognize it, but I didn't even know what color it was. I sobbed as I walked frantically through the parking lot looking for anything familiar. Finally, I ran into it. That was it! Or was it? I tried the key. It worked! Yes, that was her car! Somehow, I got myself home, but I don't remember doing it. When I was finally safe, back in my mother's kitchen, I collapsed in tears, trying to tell her what had happened, but unable to explain. It seemed like the most unbelievable, illogical story I'd ever told. How would I make sense of it, so she would understand?

But she did understand. She looked at me knowingly. "You had a panic attack," she said.

A panic attack! I thought back to that first anxiety attack I'd had in my parent's car and the anxiety that I experienced at times, but this was nothing like that. This was a whole new level of distress, a whole new universe of anxiety. Is this what my mother had been battling all those years, when we had to leave parties early or cancel our plans? This sheer, utter, mind-altering panic? Why? Why did it happen to her? Why was it happening to me?

I felt changed forever. Once you've experienced something as core-shaking as a true panic attack, it does something to you. You live with the memory like a weight attached to your back, carried wherever you go. You go to extremes to be sure you never have one again. You avoid anything you think might trigger it because you are terrified of ever being that terrified again. I began to understand why my mother closed herself off in her bedroom and stared at the TV for days at a time. It was the only way to keep the world still. If this was her life, would it become mine? Was I on the same course?

That panic attack launched me into a tailspin. Over the next weeks, panic attacks came in waves, one after the other, sometimes daily. I retreated to my room, just the way my mother had. One week became two, and two weeks became four. I lost my job. I put my acting classes on hold. I could no longer afford my rent—and even the idea of leaving my parents' house was unbearable (I would later learn that this condition has a name: agoraphobia). So, I lost my apartment, too. Going back to the city and back to work and school, or even doing something I loved, like going out dancing, was inconceivable. I lay in my childhood bed all day and all night.

When I wasn't reeling from a panic attack, I was plunged into depression. My days consisted of waking up, refusing the offer of oatmeal or a bagel from my mother, drinking some orange juice, then going back to bed until midafternoon, when I would watch talk shows for hours until the sun set. I rarely ate dinner. I barely even spoke. I felt blank, numb, as if I had no ability to form words that would make any sense to anyone. After a month of this, my mother sat at the foot of my bed and cried in frustration. She had tried everything she could think of to get me to feel better. She begged me to get up, or at least to speak to her, but I couldn't. I had nothing to say and no ability to think of something.

Every day after work, my dad came into my room and said the same thing, in the same exact words: "Did you go out today? Have you eaten? Do you feel any better? Come on, let's go for a walk." Every day, even though he knew I hadn't done and wouldn't do any of those things. There I was, lying in a bed in the same clothes I wore the day before, washed out and pale with sunken eyes, barely able to move. It was like he didn't even notice. Why the pointless questions? I turned away in disgust and stared at the wall. I certainly wasn't going to go on any walks with him.

Time rolled on, and after months of being housebound, I'd lost ten pounds I couldn't afford to lose and my depression only looked to get deeper and darker. That's when my mother found me a psychologist and demanded that I go. The idea of leaving the house seemed alien and frightening, but she insisted it was my only hope. With barely a word and no energy to protest, I let her take me.

The waiting room was brown and drab, and everyone sitting there looked drawn and sad. By the time we arrived, I was shaking badly, terrified to be out of the house and in this strange environment. The receptionist noticed my distress. She came out to talk to me. "You have to fight this," she said. "I struggled with panic attacks and depression, and I ended up housebound with agoraphobia for ten years."

I could hear her, but her words barely registered. It was as if someone had turned the light off in my brain. Logically, it was clear to me that some kind of reaction from the dental anesthetic had triggered this drastic change in me, but I also knew, deep down, that it was something more. My dad sometimes told me to shake it off, but I knew I couldn't shake it off. It was too heavy, whatever it was. There was something very wrong with me. At the same time, I didn't care. If I had to lie in bed for the rest of my life, it didn't matter. The one thing I regretted was having lost everything I'd worked so hard to get—my job, my acting classes, my new-found life in the city—but even that seemed like a distant kind of mourning and a life that I couldn't quite believe I used to live. It hung in my consciousness like a barely-remembered dream.

The psychologist peered at me through glasses that hung off the tip of his nose. He asked me questions about my life: my relationship with my mother, my father, my sister, my friends. The dental anesthesia incident didn't seem to concern him. I thought he looked like Peter Sellers as Inspector Clouseau, but less interesting. His diagnosis: I was depressed. Duh, I thought.

Then he wrote me a prescription: three Xanax daily and an antidepressant. I was just twenty years old. I remember wondering if I really needed all those pills. Surely it was something else—that dental anesthesia had ripped the top off some kind of havoc going on in my physical body. It was a trigger that set everything in motion. I had been burning the candle at both ends when I lived in the city, eating crap, barely sleeping, and that surgery threw me over the edge. And now I was paying the price. But I couldn't believe the cure was a handful of heavy medication. But I didn't have the strength or the will to argue.

I've never done well with any kind of drugs. On the Xanax, I still trembled all the time, and the antidepressant just knocked me out completely, so I couldn't move. I was still visibly shaking at our second visit, and also drenched in sweat. He upped my Xanax to four per day and changed the antidepressant to Prozac. He also decided I was probably sexually abused. No, I assured him. I was not. He brought my parents into the room to hear everything we were saying, just so someone would talk to him, because I was hardly speaking. He suggested I was angry at them, and the depression was my protest. At this point, I felt like he was just pulling ideas out of a hat…or his ass.

My so-called nervous stomach was always with me, too. I wasn't eating much but the occasional bagel here, a few bites of pasta there, and drinking orange juice, but I couldn't hold much down. The doctor said it was because of the medication, even though I hadn't been eating before. Every time I saw him, he shifted my meds—because of the trembling, or violent nightmares, or because whatever he gave me wasn't doing anything at all.

My days began to revolve around the television and its comforting drone. One night, I watched an actress on the Tonight Show. As she talked about her rise to fame, I cried silently. It was everything I wanted, right in front of me, and yet I couldn't even move from my bed. I remember pouring all the Xanax into my hand and contemplating taking them all. I put them back in the bottle, but the thought lingered in my mind.

Over the next week, the Zoloft I was taking seemed to make a little bit of difference and the doctor said we'd found the right combination: four Xanax, then a Zoloft at night. I began to function a little bit, within the confines of the house. I could get out of bed and brush my teeth and wash my hair, and I even started eating a little bit, despite my continually roiling stomach. Pretty soon, I was eating a full bowl of pasta, and even sharing the occasional pizza with my dad.

By the end of the second week on Zoloft, however, I experienced some kind of backlash, tumbling into a hole even deeper than the one I'd been in before. I began to spiral out of control, experience episodes of extreme anger, during which my blood pressure spiked. For no apparent reason, the anger would surge inside of me until I wanted to throw myself through the window. My body felt like it was screaming from the inside, but nobody could hear it. My mother took me back to the doctor. He decided we only had one option left. Shock treatment.

My parents didn't like this idea at all. I didn't either, but I also didn't care enough to protest. My mom, however, was not going to go there. She knew a woman who knew a woman who would pray over people. My mom had always believed in the power of prayer, and thought this was a far better idea than shock treatment. My mother dialed the number and handed me the phone. I took it without the energy to protest—what did I have to lose?-- and listened.

This woman, whom I had never met, prayed for me on the other end of the line with such passion, I could almost touch it. I remember her saying to me, "Now Jennifer, go rest and know that you are protected." I was happy to do what she said and go right back to bed. I didn't think much more about it.

The next morning, I awoke to the TV, still on from the night before. I heard *The Phil Donahue Show*, and with my eyes still closed, I heard Phil Donahue talking about panic attacks. A coincidence? Who knows, but it piqued my interest enough to open my eyes, sit up, and listen.

The guest was a doctor who taught cognitive therapy, and had certain exercises that he said can actually head off a panic attack by distracting the brain. He explained some of the techniques. I grabbed a pen and a piece of paper and wrote them down. He also said that people with this disorder should stay away from sugar, and that they have what was like an allergic reaction to their own serotonin. I'd never heard of this, and I didn't understand everything he was saying, but what I did understand made sense to me, especially the part about sugar. It was the first time I had ever heard anybody say anything about diet impacting a condition like this, although I had always wondered why no doctor asked me about my diet. Food seemed to me such an important part of identity, so why wouldn't it be relevant to health? When the program was over, I wrote down the name of the doctor's book, and asked my father to go out and buy it for me.

I read that book from cover to cover. I was still depressed and still taking my four daily Xanax, but something about that book made sense to me and gave me hope. It was full of ideas and solutions that had nothing to do with medication. I adopted a few suggestions from the book immediately, like eliminating sugar. I looked at the orange juice I'd been subsisting on, and realized it was pretty much pure sugar. That was out. So were the Oreos I would graze on. I asked my mom if she could fill up the refrigerator with broccoli and salad.

The book had a whole section on vitamins, which I knew nothing about. I'd never taken a vitamin in my life before reading that book, but it said that panic attacks can be linked to low levels of vitamin D and B vitamins. It recommended high dosages of B-12 in sublingual form, for the best absorption, vitamin D, and mega-doses of vitamin C. I gave my dad a list and sent him to the store. It certainly seemed like a better option than shock treatment.

A week later, I felt like a person again, still weak but alive. When my father came in my room to ask me to take a walk with him, I sat up, and then I surprised myself by agreeing. I think it took us forty minutes to get all the way around the block. I was a bucket of sweat and my heart was pounding, but my dad went slowly and kept telling me to breathe. "It's okay, see? We're walking around the block." After that, I was able to go to the store with my mom without having a panic attack, and slowly, very slowly, I began to put my life back together. Every step was small, but felt huge to me. After four months of slow but steady recovery, I thought I might be able to leave Staten Island again, and finally get on with my life!

5

back in the saddle

It took me about a year to get myself all the way back to-gether, to the point where I could have a conversation with someone without breaking out into a full soaking sweat, or talk to friends on the phone without crying, or take a ride in a car without wanting to claw my way out. During this time, my mom and I became very close. We sat around the kitchen table and I got to hear about her life and all her frustrations in a more adult way then I had in the past. I grew to know my mother in a different way than I had ever known her before. Although I'd seen all her weaknesses throughout the years regarding her health, now that I had experienced the severity of a true panic attack, I realized that my mother wasn't weak, but strong. She always tried to be better, every day, and that is not an easy road. During that time of my recovery, it truly sunk in, at a very deep level, that no matter what happened to my health, I must not let it direct my life, as I could see it had with her. "Nothing is easy," she told me. "This is the cross you bear in life, so either you accept the panic attacks and keep moving forward, or you give up. I don't want you to give up. Do not let this define you."

I realized that at times, even to this day, my mom believed in me more than I did. Because of her words, and because of my fear that I might never leave that kitchen table, I began to venture out. I kept my bag of tricks with me at all times—my Pepto-Bismol and ginger ale, with the added additions of Xanax and my cognitive therapy tricks. My favorite was the rubber band trick. I kept a rubber band around my wrist at all times, and whenever I felt like I was venturing on to that slippery slope towards panic, I would snap it. It really worked! The other one I liked was to count back from one hundred, by twos, then threes, then taking deep breaths and starting over. It's a way of stopping your mind from spiraling into panic by giving you a task or snapping yourself back into reality. Of course, I followed this technique with the insurance policy of a Xanax.

I started to take short day trips into the city, avoiding all tunnels, elevators, and crowds. I always feared an attack, and getting trapped was something I couldn't chance. The intense breathlessness and claustrophobia were paralyzing, and I would do almost anything not to wake that sleeping beast, but I feared *not* living my life even more. I took step after step, back into my independent life, and worked my way down to two Xanax per day. My stomach continued to act up, so I kept the Pepto in my purse. When I was ready, I landed a day shift waitressing job at a trendy restaurant in Soho.

One afternoon, one of the other waitresses (also a would-be actress) told me about an audition she read about in *Backstage,* an industry publication that lists auditions and casting calls. Most of them are worthless, but once in awhile, they have something real and worthwhile. I had just started back up taking acting classes at Lee Strasberg, and I was discovering that the year I'd gone through had actually improved my acting by giving me a deeper perspective into myself and the work I was studying in school. I was doing well, and feeling confident, so I figured, why not go to this open call? It would be a good experience just to audition for something.

My fellow waitress and I went to the audition together, but when we arrived, the lady in charge said we had missed the actual audition and this was a callback. However, she said we could still read if we didn't mind waiting a bit. She gave us some pages to look at, and came back half an hour later. My friend went in and came out quickly. Then it was my turn.

I was nervous, but in the context of all the fears in my life, this was nothing. I read the pages for the director. He seemed interested. He told me to wait. He wanted me to read with someone else. I did, and then he thanked me and I left.

A day later, I got a phone call. "We'd like to cast you," a woman told me. It was the lead role in an independent film that was shooting in New York that very next week! I couldn't believe what I was hearing. A movie? The *lead role?* It seemed like my big break. At the same time, however, I was worried about my health. I wasn't going to say no to this opportunity, but every day, before going to the set, I loaded up my purse with Xanax and Pepto and I put a rubber band around my wrist.

Shooting my first movie was mind-blowing. My stomach played tricks on me during the entire two-week shoot, but I applied everything I learned in acting school, and more. I remember looking around the set and thinking that, as foreign as it all felt, it also felt like home, like I'd done it a million times before. Acting allowed me to leave myself behind and step into another person's shoes for awhile. I needed to get away from myself, if only for a scene or two. I realized that acting really could be an outlet to escape everything I was dealing with, as well as a way to connect. The other people on the movie were great, and it was a "first movie" experience for many of us, so everyone was excited and grateful. Still, I always felt like my stomach was living on borrowed time, so I was relieved when it was over.

About eight months later, I was still living at home, and I had yet another waitressing job at another hip place. I was starting to get out a little with friends, going dancing at the latest clubs, but I always stayed close to the door because the crowd made me extremely nervous. I didn't want to get trapped. More than anything, I feared another panic attack. My friends would be dancing and drinking and doing the occasional party drugs, while I was popping five thousand mg of vitamin B-12 under my tongue along and Xanax just so I could stay with them. I continued with the vitamin regimen and the low-sugar diet, and I kept reading books about health—it was like a hobby, trying to unravel the link between diet and vitamins, and just being able to get out of the house. I knew it was important, but I didn't have a good grasp on it yet. I was still searching.

One night, we ventured to an after-party for some movie premiere, where I met a commercial agent. He said he worked for William Morris, and he wanted to see my resume and reel. I didn't have much of a resume, but I did have that indie movie under my belt (my pay was a copy of the film, due to me any day). I told him about the movie I was in and he said, "When you get your copy, send it to me." He introduced me to a talent agent for film, TV, and theater, also at William Morris, and he said he would be happy to look at the movie, too, once I sent it in.

For the next three weeks, I haunted the director, trying to get my copy of that tape. Finally, I got it. I started to watch it, and it was the strangest thing in the world to see myself on film. I could hardly stand to look at the screen! But I sealed up the movie in an envelope and sent it to the agents I met.

I'll never forget the night I got that phone call. I was sitting at dinner with my sister and her husband of three years. She had just told the whole family she was pregnant, and we were celebrating over dinner. The phone rang, and my mother said it was for me. It was the agent I met, Larry, calling from the William Morris agency.

I immediately lost my breath. Then I got suspicious. Was it a friend playing a joke? When I heard his familiar, raspy voice, I knew it was really him. He said he viewed the tape, and also just happened to be speaking to a very high-up executive at Miramax, who also saw the tape. He told me that the executive said, "Whoever this kid Jennifer Esposito is, she's the one to look at."

I nearly threw up. Then he asked if I would come in to meet the rest of the William Morris team next week. I must have thanked him a million times before I hung up and told my family. We had much to celebrate that night.

But I still carried the weight of fear on my back, and Xanax and Pepto in my purse. Even thinking about traveling into the city and going up to the thirty-fourth floor, where the agency was, filled me with dread. I worried about whether they would like me, but I was even more worried about that elevator. I couldn't let my anxiety stop me, but what if...what if...? The knots in my stomach made me sick. The day of the interview, I pulled myself together the best way I knew how. I tried to look "all-American," because I'd learned in acting school that I should look versatile. I put on a denim skirt and a pink mock turtleneck sweater, and pushed back my now short, brownish-red hair, trying to make myself look as presentable as possible. "You go get 'em," my mom said. I could hardly answer. I put the rubber band around my wrist, climbed into my mother's little Toyota, and set out for Manhattan.

I sang along to the radio to distract my mind and keep it from going off on a nervous tangent. The traffic was terrible. I couldn't take the bridge into the city as I usually did. I would never make it on time. I had to take the tunnel. The dreaded tunnel! I hadn't been in the tunnel in years. As I entered, I closed the car windows and turned on the fan. The car didn't have air conditioning, but I would have to make do. I sang at the top of my lungs to try to forget where I was. I felt myself starting to sweat, so I began to count calmly back from one hundred by twos and threes, breathing deeply between every number. I also popped a Xanax. The tunnel traffic started to move and I was elated when I saw the light at the other end. I had made it! But not without battle scars—my makeup was running and I knew I had sweat stains under my arms. Still, I had to get there. I no longer cared how I looked. I had one goal in mind: Get to the William Morris office.

Finally, I was there. I looked up at the tall building and hesitated. Then I said to myself, "Okay. You have two choices. You get in that elevator and get up there, or you stay down here and go home and die in Staten Island." I pushed ahead. I had read in an article somewhere that Julia Roberts listened to her headphones to psych herself up before an audition and drown out the world around her. I needed to do that at that moment, so out came my earphones and I plugged myself in. I stepped up to the elevator and Whitney Houston's voice poured into my ears: "I'm every woman!" It felt right for the moment—the anthem I needed. With my mascara running down my face, sweating, hair messed up, humming madly to myself, I stepped into the elevator and pressed thirty-four. I watched the floors go by as sweat trickled down my sides and back and ran under the band of my denim skirt. Then the doors opened, and there I was, on the thirty-fourth floor, with the big William Morris sign staring me in the face. I made it.

Shaking just a little, I walked into the office. There were two other girls sitting there waiting for meetings, too. One was a beautiful, fair-skinned, elegant Marilyn Monroe look-alike. The other girl was a beauty as well. They looked at me like I must be lost, and I admit I felt lost at that moment. I felt like getting back on the elevator and going back home. I didn't look like those girls. Not even a little. They were elegant. Not sweating, obviously not on the edge of vomiting. They had beautiful skin and beautiful hair, and they both looked more serene than I think I've ever felt in my life. But I sat down. If I could make it this far, then I could go all the way. I focused on Whitney Houston's voice, and although with every passing moment, a new thought arose that I should get up and run away, I wouldn't let myself. I stayed in my seat.

When the receptionist finally called me into a back room, I opened the huge boardroom doors to find seven well-dressed executive types sitting at a big table. I felt like a little girl in the principal's office. They asked me some questions, but I don't remember much about it. I do remember that I could have cut the judgment in the air with a knife. I didn't think they liked me. When it was over, I thanked everyone for taking the time to meet with me, and I got out of that building as fast as I could, embarrassed, but at the same time, elated. I did it! By the time I got home, I was drained and exhausted, but proud of myself. Just doing it—that had been my goal, no matter what they thought of me.

The next day, Larry called me personally.

"Honestly, kid, some of the agents didn't get it." I knew that by "it" he meant me. "But you know what? I get it. And I know you're going to work. I'm going to take you on personally, on one condition. I also want you to meet with a manager and the commercial agency, so I have some backup with getting you out there. Deal?"

We had a deal. I never forgot those people in that room who didn't get me. They only fueled my fire. I wanted to prove them wrong. I would become what I knew I could become, health problems be damned. All I needed was one person to believe in me, and thankfully, I had found one. I would become what I knew I could be: A working actress.

AT LONG LAST, I moved out of my parent's home again. I found a 250-square-foot, rent-stabilized apartment in a fifth floor walk-up in the West Village. It was so small that I could almost touch both sides of the wall when standing in the center, but I didn't care. I loved it there. It was all mine. I had a hot plate and a mini fridge, and that was all I needed. I cooked my meals on the hot plate and sat on my bed, which was also my dining room. It was pure bliss. I auditioned a lot, and got small jobs here and there. Sometimes, I did plays for no money, but I didn't care. I loved acting and building a career for myself.

Meanwhile, a friend's family owned a French restaurant up the street from where I lived, and I went there often because I could eat for free, and the jobs I was getting at that time weren't paying me very much. It was a whole new way of eating for me—steamed artichokes, Niçoise salads, and a lot of omelettes. Dates often took me to restaurants, too, and I began to appreciate the New York food scene in a whole new way, beyond the pasta and bagels I'd been eating for the past year. This sparked a new level of commitment in my love affair with food. I wasn't hoarding sugary cereal or pigging out on pizza anymore. I began to appreciate different flavors. I ate more vegetables, meat, and cheeses from all over the world. I bought day-old bread at a discount from Balducci's, an Italian market in my neighborhood, and topped it with a tomato, olive oil, and salt. It was simple and cheap, but it was my favorite meal (and still is).

For two years, I auditioned, worked, and had some much-needed fun in the city. I was a working actress, and my rent was so cheap that, eventually, I didn't have to wait tables anymore. When my acting teacher told me there was nothing else he could teach me and I just had to get out there and go for it, I took his advice. I always had my Xanax and I was always ready for my sensitive stomach to act up, but I was managing things. Then I got an audition for what would be the biggest role of my career thus far.

My agent sent me on an audition to be a series regular on a comedy that filmed in NYC, but they told me I needed to work on my comedy. I'd been studying drama for so long in a school that looked down its nose at comedy, so I'd never really honed my comedy skills. But this was a job—a good job—this was *Spin City*, and it had a great cast. It would mean money and a lot of good exposure. I was even more anxious when I found that I would be reading with the lead of the show for my callback.

I watched episode after episode of *Seinfeld* to get my brain into comedy mode, and on the day of the audition, I was so nervous, I was shaking, but I tried not to think about that. I met Michael and we read the scene together. My plan: Do the scene exactly the way Elaine would have done it on *Seinfeld*. No joke, this was my strategy—and it worked! Everyone in the room laughed. I was just happy to get through the audition without having a panic attack or throwing up. The next day, I got the call: The job was mine. I was going to be a series regular.

This was one of the best jobs I'd ever had. Everyone in the cast was welcoming and talented and so nice. The show was shot in New York in front of a live audience, so it felt familiar to me, like theater. I loved every day, but it also fueled my confidence and ambition. I was ready to fly. I was booking films and doing them on the television show's summer hiatus.

When I got cast in *Summer of Sam,* directed by Spike Lee, I felt like I'd taken my career to a new level. The director called me himself to ask if I wanted a role in his movie.

"Yes!" I tried not to scream it, and then I thanked him with everything I had. I hung up the phone and cried my eyes out. This was the kind of work I'd been dreaming about and working towards in all those years of acting classes. Then I realized I would need the first two weeks off from season 3 of *Spin City* in order to film it. It would work out. It had to work out.

The producers said no.

I couldn't believe I wouldn't be able to keep a job that I loved and was grateful for and do this dream movie! My agent tried everything to make things work, but they wouldn't budge. The role was given to another actress. I was absolutely heartbroken. I didn't know how I could go back to the show I once loved under this condition. Then I was given a miraculous second chance—Spike Lee offered me a different role in the movie. I would only need two days off. Again, the TV show said no—I wasn't even allowed to take two days off! I was flabbergasted. I realized I was in a contract, but it was only two rehearsal days and I was resolved to make it work. I had to do this movie! I begged the director to change my filming days and take half the money he was offering. Finally, he agreed, and I managed to do it.

The shoot was extraordinary. It was everything I thought it would be, and more. I had time to really dive into my role and get lost in it. It was challenging, but I loved every minute of it, and it made me want to do more movies. The whole experience took its toll on my relationship with my job, however, and I felt like I let people at the TV show down. Towards the end of filming season three, I became terribly ill. The year before, on Christmas break, I'd been bedridden for two weeks with the flu that the entire crew seemed to have, and I certainly knew what a sinus infection was because I'd already had many, but this was something different—something insidious and new. I broke out in sores all over my face and body. I had a fever of 103 for four days, and incredible pain in my lower back and right side. I was also weaker than I'd ever been. I finally went to the doctor, who did blood work and found that my liver was severely inflamed. He said it wasn't hepatitis. It seemed to be some sort of liver virus.

That would be the first time that anyone ever even suggested that my being sick might not be real, or was just an excuse for wanting to leave the show. That certainly wasn't the case. I loved my job, but I could barely get out of bed. I recovered, but sadly parted ways with the show after that. I was so grateful for my time there and everything I learned, but it was time to move on.

My health continued to go up and down, and I continued in my quest to learn everything I could about the things I could do to improve my health. I exercised whenever I could, ate the foods I thought were healthy, and read all the books on the latest health fads, and I applied everything that made sense to me. I was open to any new approach to health, and adopted anything that made me feel better. I liked the idea of holistic care because so many doctors had been unable to help me by this point, and I wanted to be able to help myself. Frankly, I probably would have gone to a witch doctor at this point if I thought it would help me! I saw a chiropractor for the lower back pain, a general practitioner for the stomach issues and headaches, massage therapists for my fatigue and stress, and then, one day, a friend suggested I try applied kinesiology. I researched this, and learned that applied kinesiologists used muscle testing to determine which foods and other substances were allergenic or damaging to a particular person. Maybe I was eating or doing something that was hurting me. I thought it was certainly worth a try.

The applied kinesiologist came to my house casually dressed, not like a doctor at all. He had a peaceful vibe. He looked around my apartment and told me to gather up all the things I eat from my refrigerator and cabinets, along with all the facial cleansers, shampoos, and other personal products I use. I set a mound of things on the couch. First, he had me hold a bottle of shampoo, and then hold out my right arm. He pushed lightly on my arm. Strangely, I wasn't able to resist the push! I figured it was some kind of fluke, but then he put some soap in my hand, and I had no trouble holding my arm against his push. He said that when my arm could be easily pushed down, that meant my body didn't like that item or was almost, you could say, allergic. About half my personal products caused my arm to go down! How could I possibly be reacting to so many things? I thought maybe my arm was getting tired, so I switched arms, but the results remained the same. Then we started on the food.

Almost every food we tried caused my arm to go down with the slightest push. Even he was shocked at how many foods I was reacting against. He said it meant I had quite a few food allergies. This made me skeptical—how could I really be allergic to all the food in my kitchen? He recommended I get rid of everything I reacted against, but that was almost everything. I couldn't imagine what would be left to eat. And could I afford to just throw away half my personal products? It was just too much to take in at once. I decided to think about it, but I wasn't going to throw everything away. It just seemed too rash.

But it didn't mean I had stopped searching for remedies to all that ailed me. Another friend recommended yoga, which seemed to help calm my mind and my stomach. I practiced as much as I could. I also did hard workouts to stay in shape because I was well on my way as an up-and-coming actress, and I had to stay in shape and somehow find ways to stay healthy. This constant searching just became part of my life.

6

my public success,
my private war

$\mathcal{U}$pon *Summer of Sam's* release, directors began to consider me for bigger and bigger roles. I was flying back and forth to Los Angeles frequently, but I paid a price for it. I always loaded up on my Xanax, Dramamine, and ginger ale, but flights were incredibly uncomfortable. Every flight, I feared a panic attack in the cramped airplane cabin, knowing I wouldn't be able to escape for hours.

I was getting beat up by the business as well. I was disillusioned as I came to realize that acting was, first and foremost, a business that operates according to some very specific rules. I realized that talent, acting chops, and individuality weren't valued nearly as much as generic, all-American good looks, youth, and the latest box office tally. I kept pushing on through some very rough patches to make a career for myself, and it was working, but it took a toll on my soul as well as my body. My panic attacks began to recur more regularly, and my nervous stomach issues increased. I started to get severe headaches followed by severe sinus infections again. Of course, my doctors always treated these with course after course of antibiotics, and when those didn't work, steroids.

I've always had olive skin with a yellow tinge, but my skin began to get sallow, a duller, unattractive yellow color that makeup artists often complained about. They had a terrible time trying to match my tone, or make it less yellow with gray. It looked unnatural, and I got labeled as "difficult" among the makeup artists, as if I had some control over the color of my skin. Another strange thing that constantly plagued the wardrobe people was my changing size, as if my body was swelling and then deflating according to a will of its own. I'd always owned "bloated clothes" and "unbloated clothes," but try explaining that to wardrobe! On swollen days, I often turned down social events. I couldn't bear to walk the red carpet and be judged by the media. No thanks. So I hid away, which didn't help my career. Publicists and managers often directed me to go to this or that event, present this award or make an appearance, but I frequently said no because I was afraid that my health might play tricks on me, and to be judged when I already wasn't feeling well didn't seem appealing. Then, as I felt I was foiling my own career, I became more and more depressed. Finally, I decided to seek out a therapist on my own, not because a doctor was telling me to, but because I felt like maybe I could use some calm and objective advice.

My therapist was a sweet, kind woman who believed in the mind/body connection. I worked with her for about two years, and she inspired my interest in the many ways that the mind and body are connected. I didn't know what it was like to be free of pain, nausea, depression, and panic attacks. It had all become "normal" for me, especially because that was my mother's life as well as mine. It was my cross to bear, as she had once told me. Everyone has problems, right? But I did read many of the books my therapist recommended, and I began to learn more about my body and adopt new strategies, hoping to feel just a little bit better.

One of the books in particular struck me. It said that every organ is attached to an emotion, and your entire emotional history lies in your cells. That idea fascinated me. Therapy helped me work out a lot of things. We discussed my past, and she helped me begin to understand that my current health situation maybe wasn't so normal, and maybe there was a deep bodily connection between my health and my emotions. I remember reading a line in another book she suggested for me: "Your health is a direct manifestation of your thoughts." That one really startled me, and I couldn't help wondering if it was true. On the one hand, you can change your thoughts, so that sounded like I could change my health. On the other hand, it also implied I'd brought it all on myself. That thought discouraged me. Maybe it was all my fault. Maybe I really was my own worst enemy. Still, I couldn't swallow that completely, and my searching continued. I went to healers who claimed they could bring light into my body through their hands. I went to chakra cleansing classes, and even to past life regression people, all in hopes of finding some peace with my health. I tried a vegan diet. I tried a macrobiotic diet. When something worked, I kept it. When something didn't work, I moved on.

Through all this, I was continuing to work on set, doing a lot of movies and appearing on various TV shows. I was busy, and it was awesome, but my health issues always loomed. Life on the set can be tough at times. For example, one morning, on the set of a movie I was doing, I was walking to the makeup room. I had my pre-mixed makeup in my hand. I was tired. We'd been filming late the night before, and what can I say?—it was 5 a.m.! I passed a group of producers talking amongst themselves and I didn't pay much attention because they seemed pretty occupied with their conversation. It didn't seem like my place to talk to them—I was always a little bit fearful about saying something stupid or doing something wrong, so I wanted to just do my job and go home. I vaguely remember picking my head up long enough to offer a small smile. They nodded, and I kept walking.

Midday, I got a call from my agent.

"Jennifer. Are you happy on set?"

"Um…yes? Why?"

"The producers called and said you don't seem happy. They said you didn't even say hello to them this morning."

I thought: Seriously? Happy? Am I happy? It was 5:00 a.m.! I never meant to be rude at all, but this is how it can be on set. Every move you make might be scrutinized, and any suggestion of an attitude will be noted. Every pimple and every line will be counted. Everything you say, do, even your expression will be up for interpretation. The set is not a place for being tired, for having health issues, for sadness, headaches, or stupid questions. Add to that the stress of having to perform and be great. Sets can be amazing environments, but they can also be hard environments where the judgment is constant. When you're not feeling your best, it can be tough.

AFTER 9/11, I began to despise planes even more than usual. I decided to get a place in L.A., while still keeping my place in New York. Like many people, I was shaken by how I now saw the world after that horrific occurrence. I needed a place in L.A. so I wouldn't have to travel back and forth so much. A place that felt safe. I found L.A. to be overwhelming and I only knew a few people there. To ease my heart a bit, I brought home a Golden Retriever puppy, part of a litter from a veterinarian who bred his two Goldens. Frankie Beans came with me to many sets, and sat on many cold bathroom floors with me while I was sick. He was, and still is, my very best friend. He has always known when I was feeling badly, and he always had the most hopeful expression on his face, like he was trying to will away my pain.

I had learned to keep my health issues to myself, for the most part—only Frankie Beans knew how bad it was—until I got the movie of a lifetime: Crash. I was cast playing the detective partner of Don Cheadle's character. The script was one of the best things I'd ever read. I was beyond excited…until I realized I was going to have to be naked. *On camera.* On a big screen in movie theaters. My body, right there for all the world to see.

Usually, when you come to a sex scene or a nude scene in a script, you can modify it to the level that makes you comfortable by talking to the director about it, and what you will and won't do goes into your contract, but, for this movie, the naked scene was necessary. The director thought it was important that my character be naked because it makes her vulnerable in the scene. From a purely artistic standpoint, I completely agreed with him. But personally? Yikes! I had one month before filming the scene, and so I felt incredible pressure to look and, more importantly, feel as comfortable as possible. I didn't want to be worried about my body and not have my mind on the scene at hand. The Atkins Diet was the diet of the moment—protein and vegetables only, no carbs. I decided that, for one month, I would cut out all breads, pasta, and sweets. It was hard, but I did it.

I was determined not to cheat. I also signed up with the best personal trainer there was. I began to live on hard-boiled eggs for breakfast, lots of salads, vegetables, and tons of protein. For dessert, I had fruit, or the occasional sorbet. The change was amazing—I was full of energy and my stomach bloat completely disappeared. I began to get leaner and the swelling subsided, too. My whole lower body looked different. I think if I hadn't been feeling so focused on the part, the changes might have been more obvious to me at the time, or I might have made some connection to my new diet, but I just thought I was losing weight because I was dieting and exercising regularly.

The day of the shoot, I was nervous, but I felt good and tried to forget about my insecurities. Don and I both laughed at the awkwardness of the whole situation, and on one of the breaks, he admitted he'd been dieting and working out, too—he had the same worries about exposing his body as I did. His honesty relaxed me. We finished the scene and we were both relieved. The craft services girl walked by us with fried chicken, and we both gladly took a giant piece. The scene was over, and so was the deprivation! That night, to celebrate, I went out to meet some friends, and we had pizza and some kind of double-chocolate something for dessert. The next day, I was sick as a dog. It was time to start shooting again. My call time was later in the day, so I stayed in bed for as long as I could. The headaches were back and I felt like I had a terrible hangover. I was nauseous and my stomach sent me to the bathroom every twenty minutes.

About ninety minutes before my ride was scheduled to pick me up and bring me in, it started in earnest. My nervous stomach was taking no prisoners and letting me know exactly who was boss. I couldn't stop running to the bathroom. Then I contracted a fever. I felt like I'd been poisoned. I remember being so weak that all I could do was lie on the bathroom floor with Frankie Beans at my side. I called my manager immediately and said the dreaded words I'd hoped I'd never have to say: "I can't move." She told me it was probably food poisoning, or the flu that was going around the set. The producers sent a doctor to my house—something they had to do for insurance reasons. The doctor was shocked at how weak I was. He said I was so dehydrated that my blood pressure had dropped dangerously low. He wouldn't let me go to work. What?! Up until that day, I'd never missed a single day of work since that major illness during the *Spin City* days. I couldn't believe this was happening, on one of the best projects I'd ever had the honor to be a part of.

I was devastated beyond words. The doctor hooked up my bed to support two IVs so he could rehydrate me. The producers weren't happy, of course, but they did have many people dropping from the flu, and they figured I'd gotten whatever was going around as well.

It was just two days before Christmas. I was due back in New York. Even though I now spent most of the year in L.A., I couldn't bear living there full-time. I'm a New Yorker at heart and I'd needed my regular NYC fix, so I always kept my apartment. I wanted so badly to get home, so I nursed myself as well as I could. I ate nothing but chicken soup and crackers, and loaded up on Imodium AD Extra Strength and Xanax to get me through the five-hour plane ride. When I was back in New York, I was so glad to collapse and finally get some rest. I began to feel better and I wondered if stress had caused the entire episode.

I got through the holidays, not at my best but doing well enough to join in my family's holiday festivities. I was due back in L.A. five days after New Year's to shoot my remaining scene. I was still exhausted and my stomach was still acting up, but I thought the bagels and crackers I was living on must be helping. I went to a restaurant around the corner from my apartment a few days before I had to be back in L.A., and suddenly, the nausea and the urgency to find a bathroom swept over me again. I ran home, and six hours later, I was in the emergency room. I was sick for hours. The Imodium I usually relied on wasn't working. I became so dehydrated that I was taken to a room and kept for observation. The doctors poked and prodded me while I stared at a TV that was playing repeats of *Spin City*. The doctor who had his finger up my rectum asked me if that was me on the television. I kid you not.

My mom and dad came to the hospital as soon as they heard, but the blood work didn't show a thing. My liver enzymes were very high, but they decided I probably had food poisoning. Again? And for an entire month? I told the doctors that didn't make sense to me. Just a month ago, the exact thing had happened to me. Something wasn't right. All I got was, *Sorry, that's our diagnosis.*

I went home and stared in the mirror. My skin was sallow and yellow, and I was so weak, I couldn't imagine flying back to L.A. I called my therapist and she agreed to see me. I was a bundle of tears. I told her about my health issues and how I had to be back in L.A. in two days. Was it stress? Was I doing this to myself? I needed to know! Although she believed in the mind-body connection, and she did believe stress was playing a part, she also thought something else was going on. What a relief that was to me! She sent me to a gastro-enterologist the next day.

The gastroenterologist was at least focused on my stomach. He took more blood and prescribed four doses of Pepto-Bismol daily, and put me on an antibiotic. He believed I had some kind of bacteria. I did what he said, but by the next day, I was in severe pain and panicking about not being able to go back and finish the best movie that I ever made. My mother begged me to just let the movie go, to call the producers and tell them I wasn't coming back, that my health was more important. I refused. I had to go back! But there I was, lying on the bathroom floor in sheer agony.

The next day, just as I was beginning to think I might have to call them after all and throw away everything I wanted so badly, the producers called to tell me that the shoot had moved to a few weeks later. Then I found out it was because the director had had a heart attack, but was okay. I was worried and sad for him, but also so relieved that I had a little more time to get myself together. That night, I ended up back in the hospital. They purged me of all the Pepto-Bismol because they said it was backing up my system, causing pain. When I awoke the next morning, my sister called to tell me she'd got me in to see this supposedly amazing gastroenterologist. I was ready to try anything—I had to get in shape to get back on the set!

This new doctor was touted as one of the best. He was a kind man who believed in incorporating both eastern and western medical techniques, including acupuncture and stress management. Once I got into the exam room with him, I broke down into tears. I explained that my stomach issues had plagued me for my entire life, and now they were actually interfering with my career. I begged him to help me. I wanted to set up a colonoscopy for the next day, but I was so sore that I couldn't bear the thought of it. The doctor said it sounded like my nerves were wreaking havoc on my body. He sent me home with a stomach relaxer and some mega-doses of acidophilus. He said it would help regulate the good and bad bacteria in the gut. He also wanted me to meditate every day, for my nerves. I'd had other people tell me I should meditate, but I never thought it would have anything to do with my stomach.

With this doctor's help, I made it back to L.A. and managed to finish the movie without having another health breakdown. After I finished, I went back to New York to get the colonoscopy. I still wasn't feeling well, but I liked what that doctor had done for me so far, so I wanted to give him the chance to find out more.

The day of the exam, my mom took me for the test. A very sweet nurse took me into the exam room, trying to comfort me and minimize my fears. She told me to get completely undressed and put on a paper robe. I did what she said, feeling ridiculous in the flimsy paper. She told me to lie on my left side facing the wall, with my knees up. Then she asked for my arm, where she put in an IV with a mild sedative. I began to relax and I even closed my eyes as the doctor came in and asked if I was okay. I nodded drowsily. I barely felt a thing, until the doctor said, "Oh my. Jennifer, can you look at the screen?"

I craned my neck around, and there was the inside of my colon. Not something you see every day.

"Do you see all those little pockets?" he said, pointing to the screen. I nodded groggily. "Those aren't supposed to be there. This is pretty unusual." After it was over, I got dressed and sat down with him in his office. He said I had something that looked like *Clostridium difficile* colitis, often called *C. diff.* This is a very dangerous bacteria in the colon that takes over, often after too many courses of antibiotics, but it's unusual to see in a young person. It's usually confined to older people, often in nursing homes, who don't have strong immune systems. He put me on a medication called Flagyl and a stomach tranquilizer. I went home, weak as can be, and my mom made me a bagel and some tea to calm my stomach before taking my medication.

By the end of the day, I couldn't walk. I would stand up to go to the bathroom and my knees would give out completely. The pain in my stomach was astounding and my head felt like it was in the clouds. I couldn't think clearly, and then I could barely form sentences. My mother didn't like how I looked so she went back to my apartment with me. When my dad came by to check on us, he found me collapsed on the floor on the way back to my bedroom. He called my name and asked me if I could hear him, if I was okay. I could hear him, but I felt like I was slipping away. I couldn't speak. I knew I was in trouble, but there wasn't a thing I could do to help myself. My parents rushed me back to the hospital.

Once there, the nurses propped me up and gave me a dose of Benadryl. The doctors believed I was having some kind of allergic reaction. Once again, my blood pressure was shockingly low. They admitted me, and then immediately quarantined me, to prevent the *C. diff* from spreading, as it's highly contagious. For four days, I lay there, quarantined, getting Flagyl pumped through my veins to kill off the *C. diff*. Nurses came into my room wearing what looked like hazmat suits. I was either completely out of it, or sobbing uncontrollably. I spent a lot of time wondering why this was happening to me. I didn't have an answer. Nobody seemed to have an answer. Finally, after one more colonoscopy to confirm that the *C. diff* had cleared, they let me go home. My instructions: No antibiotics unless absolutely necessary!

Why was my gut bacteria so off? I had been on plenty of antibiotics in my life, but I couldn't believe that I was the only one. Why did I get this *C. diff*? The doctor's only answer: "You probably contracted it from someone." Yuck. I assumed he was right, and tried to forget about the whole thing. One more bizarre and seemingly random health crisis to add to the list.

7

one step forward,
two steps back

I've always been someone who enjoys having plenty of alone time, but that was pushed to the limit as my health issues became more unpredictable. I began to close the world out more and more, for fear of another embarrassment, another panic attack, another stomach attack. Just as my career was doing so well, my health was incredibly up and down. When I felt well, I was a vivacious, take-life-by-its-heels type of person, and I loved going out, traveling and having fun. When my health worsened, I became withdrawn, frightened, and depressed, and I felt hopeless. If that wasn't enough stress, I'd then get mad at myself for letting my health get to me. At that point, I was also becoming disillusioned with my career. I was also becoming disillusioned with the people I was dating, and the people I was surrounded with as well. Everybody seemed to want to be somebody else, instead of just being who they actually were. I was never very good at dating and the truth is, basically all the people I was around were all very into their careers, first and foremost. Of course, I understood this because I'm in the business, too. To have any success, you have to be somewhat self-obsessed. You have to be concerned with how you look, how you act, personally and professionally, what color your hair is, what you should wear to the next event, who you work with, and how you express yourself. It's all up for constant criticism and judgment, and one wrong move can ruin your career. To really make a career in the business I chose, you have to be ready, willing, and able to drop everything and everyone if that dream job suddenly shows up.

I understand it. I also realized that it's not an environment that fosters healthy relationships, and the whole notion of constant obsession with myself and my career began to make me very unhappy. I often felt sad beyond words about some of the things I saw and experienced. We all have to face our disillusionments. At the same time, it was the only work I knew how to do, and although it hasn't been easy, it has been wonderful at times. But the older I got, the more I began to realize that I just wasn't willing to be that person who would give up everything else to be successful.

This was a tough pill to swallow. All my life, acting was all I'd ever wanted to do, but I was facing the realities of the business, who I was becoming, and the fact that I didn't know how well they fit together anymore. I longed to do something that could make a difference in people's lives on a more personal level. I had spent years dedicated to acting and my health woes. I craved giving something back, but I had no idea what or how. I decided I needed some time off. When my friend Joanna suggested that we both desperately needed a vacation, I agreed. Although I was worried about my health and how I would handle it, I loaded up with Imodium, Xanax, crackers, and ginger ale, and we boarded a plane for Italy for some much needed fun.

We spent two amazing weeks wandering around and eating everything and making many Italian friends. Surprisingly, I felt great. My health was what it was, but I felt like I just letting it be what it was while trying to enjoy myself regardless—embracing the moment, the food, and the carefree existence, even if it was a little forced at times. I was eating pasta, bread, salad, cheese, fish, meat, everything! The food was so fresh and tasted amazing, like nothing I had been eating in the States. The bread was freshly baked, the pasta was hand-rolled right before eating, the vegetables were freshly picked from gardens, and everything was homemade and *real*. I had a few minor stomach issues, but nothing like I had at home. I was on a steady supply of Xanax to keep the panic at bay, but I felt better than I had in a long time. But the problem with vacations is that they don't last forever. As soon as I got back to New York (and back to my regular diet), I felt worse than ever. My stomach flared up again, I became weak, and depression crept back into my life. I went back to the gastroenterologist, who told me that I was too high-strung and nervous, and I needed to meditate. He also thought I might have gotten a parasite while vacationing.

"In Italy?" I asked. We'd stayed in nice places and eaten the freshest foods. A parasite seemed like a reach, but I said okay to the antibiotic he prescribed. (By the way, this is the same doctor who told me, "No antibiotics unless absolutely necessary." A phantom parasite must have been necessary.)

It frustrated me to no end to feel so sick again because I knew I couldn't go back to L.A. until I felt better. Frankie Beans was waiting for me in L.A. and I missed him so much. He always brought me a level of comfort I didn't have with anyone else, and I felt a great need for him at that time in my life. He was the one and only unwavering aspect of my existence. He was comfort and all non-judgmental, unconditional love I needed, in one package, complete with fluffy, wagging tail. He was the one who sat on many a cold bathroom floor with me, and never cared what I was wearing or how I looked or how well my last movie or TV show had done.

In the meantime, as I was recovering, I was on my way to drop off a stool sample at the doctor's office (isn't my life glamorous?), and I saw a Bernese mountain dog in the window of a pet store. She was three months old. I walked in, told the owner I'd be back in twenty minutes, and dropped off that sample. It was one of those moments when I thought my life couldn't get any more embarrassing, so I decided I needed give myself a present, as a way to make up in some small measure for everything I had endured. But she wasn't that small! To get another pup seemed like a great idea at that moment. If one dog was good, two would be even better, and Frankie Beans could have a companion when I wasn't around. I could barely walk myself home because I was so weak from all the medications I was on, but somehow I managed to get all twenty pounds of her back to my apartment. I named her Betty Boop. When I was feeling better, Betty Boop and I drove back to L.A., and I introduced the two dogs. They loved each other immediately, and my happiness doubled.

Back in L.A., I began to feel a little bit better. I started going out more, and demanded more of myself. I was determined to take my life back from illness. I started doing more yoga to calm myself down (as everyone kept suggesting), and then I saw another *Oprah* episode about staying positive and being grateful. I liked this strategy. I was grateful for many things. I tried to remember this every day and incorporate more positivity into my life. I even made a vision board for myself, with images of what I wanted for my future: a true purpose, good health, a loving partner. I felt my constant high-level anxiety beginning to ebb, but I still felt like something was off, just under the surface. Even when nothing was wrong that I could exactly put my finger on, I still felt like something was wrong.

My latest symptom was extreme backaches. I didn't think this could be related to any of my other issues, but the pain was agonizing. At the same time, I was getting recurring urinary tract infections. I went to doctor after doctor, but all anyone ever came up with was that it must be from bacteria. There was that word again. Bacteria. The word made my skin crawl, and it just didn't make sense. Where was I contracting all this bacteria? One doctor told me I might have kidney stones since my kidney and liver both seemed inflamed for no apparent reason. The doctor gave me 200 Bactrim and told me to take one a day since I was prone to urinary tract infections. He said to just continue. Forever?

"Forever," he said. Even though my gastroenterologist had warned me against antibiotics? I took them for a week, then threw them away.

Again, I began to investigate on my own. I incorporated fresh unsweetened cranberry juice and cranberry herbal supplements. I read every self-help book I could find about healing your past, healing through positive thinking, healing in any way, shape, or form. I tried so hard to link my stomach problems, panic attacks, chronic sinus infections, and now, backaches together, but all the books attributed different emotions to each of those things. I couldn't bring it all together. Where was the common thread? Or was I just born to be broken?

I wanted to change my whole life and start all over again with a new body—one that worked. I thought I could maybe leave the business for a bit, take a break, start over—but at that point, I didn't have the slightest idea how to do that. I longed to just enjoy life, like I had in Italy. I wanted to be a normal person. Maybe even, dare I say it, find someone to spend my life with? But finding someone to love, who loved me, in this lonely city of Los Angeles was seeming more and more impossible every day.

Then I met someone and accepted a date. I should have noticed the red flags from the beginning—actually, they were more like an entire marching band squad of red flags—but I ignored them because, honestly, I didn't think the relationship was really going to go anywhere. He was funny, smart, cocky, arrogant, and a master manipulator. I didn't necessarily find him that attractive, but I figured that I could enjoy his sense of humor and nonsense for a while. One date became two, two dates became four. We had fun, but he also had a mean, cold side. His personality could flip on a dime, but that kind of behavior was familiar to me. I'd spent plenty of time walking on eggshells in my childhood home as well as on certain sets, so I quickly learned my role in the relationship and went forward accordingly.

But the relationship was about him and what he needed, and nothing else. I was a non-issue. I became sidelined from my life, my needs, and my health. I became very sad and I felt very alone, but I stayed in the relationship. It wasn't all bad all the time, so I figured this was just my lot, and I took the good with the bad, even though the bad was extremely bad. That's when I discovered cooking and baking.

I FOUND A sense of peace when I was in the kitchen. Food was a comfort to me. In my childhood, food had always brought people together, so at first I used it to please my un-pleasable boyfriend. I cooked for him constantly, in an effort to keep things peaceful, but also in an effort to soothe myself and take my mind off this unhealthy relationship I found myself in. I began to devour cookbooks and cooking and baking magazines, and watched the Food Network incessantly. I made everything from soups to cakes, and even my own pizza. I was so immersed in the whole allure of cooking that I even started checking out culinary schools. I felt peaceful when I was cooking. It was a form of meditation for me.

One day, while I was making some elaborate dinner, I was watching *Oprah* and one of the guests mentioned that he gave lectures at a place called Agape—at least, that was my understanding of it. I was fascinated by the man, who was full of words I needed to hear at that moment. I thought it might be interesting to go to this place and hear more. I decided to go to Agape. I had no idea that it was a church.

With the relationship getting to be more of a roller coaster and more abusive in my eyes, I set out the next weekend to go to this place called Agape. I arrived at a large auditorium filled with hundreds of people, all waiting for the reverend to speak. The reverend?

What had I gotten myself into? Was it some kind of a cult? But as long as I'd driven all that way, I figured I might as well see what it was all about. As I waited for the lecture, or the church service, or whatever it was going to be, I didn't know what I wanted or needed to hear. I just knew I needed something.

The mass-like lecture began with a song and readings from all different types of books. It wasn't religious, exactly, but it was positive and inspiring and spiritual. Everyone around me was singing and smiling and looked genuinely happy. It felt unreal to me. I don't think I'd ever been in the presence of that many happy people at one time. There was a feeling of peaceful energy in the room, and as I looked at the faces around me, the smiles seemed to come from within the people, like their souls were smiling.

Next, the entire auditorium did a meditation together. We were asked to close our eyes and listen to our own breathing and "let it be." I took a couple of deep breaths. Let it be. Whatever that meant. I opened my eyes and looked around. Everyone was doing it! They were all just sitting quietly, just *being*. Weird. I expected to see at least a few people looking around or scoffing or rolling their eyes, but no—I was the only one peeking, the only one not absorbed in the moment. I closed my eyes again and took a few more breaths, and said to myself, "Just be, Jennifer. Just be." Thoughts flew through my brain, and then one nanosecond of huge, blissful, reverberating silence. Silence in my brain was something I had never experienced. I never knew it could exist. I was a thinker and it seemed as though my thoughts were always raring to go. This unexpected moment of pure silence was pure bliss to me. These people definitely knew something I most certainly did not, and I wanted to learn more.

Then the reverend began to talk. He had a joyful demeanor but a no-nonsense way of speaking that I appreciated. This wasn't religious and it wasn't New Agey mumbo-jumbo, either. One thing really rang true, and I've never forgotten it: "Stop trying to make things the way you want them or the way you perceive they should be. Instead, see things the way they actually are. As ugly and as beautiful. Therein lies your freedom. Therein lies your answer. And let it be."

Tears began to flow down my cheeks. I didn't know exactly what that meant fully, but it rang true to me. Let it be. Could I really do that? It sounded so simple, so honest. Not like giving up, but accepting reality for what it was, rather than what I wanted it to be or thought it should be. To stop trying to adjust everything, and just see it for what it actually was. To stop denying and constantly fighting. What a concept—to stop trying and just be who I was and where I was in my life at that point. I had been trying to make everything in my world into something better or different than it really was. My career, my health, my relationship. I decided right then to do nothing about any aspect of my life for awhile. I would just let it be so it could unfold, so I could really look at it and see what was true.

I went home feeling at peace. It was a strange feeling for me. I'm a do-er by nature, but when I got back, all I knew was: *Do nothing.* Within days, my relationship hit an all-time low, and within a week, it was over. Abruptly, rudely, and with the exact callousness that I'd come to expect from him, but this time, I did nothing but agree to end it. I didn't fight it, or try to talk him out of it, or try to make it something it wasn't. Instead of trying to fix him, fix me, fix the relationship, fix my career, instead of trying to label anything or work on anything, I decided to let it be and honestly see what my life really was.

The relationship was a hard one, but I learned many things. It opened up a world of cooking and baking that I didn't know I loved so much. It also made me painfully aware of how ugly my own self-obsession was. I was up-close-and-personal with one of the most self-obsessed humans you could imagine, and it made me take a good look at myself. I didn't want to be anything like that, and more than ever, it made me want to find some other purpose in life besides being an actor. This crazy ride also led me to Agape, where I learned the value of meditation, a gift I still carry with me as I still try to practice it every day.

As I moved on with my life, cooking became more than a hobby. It was pure pleasure. I loved nothing more than having five-course dinner parties that went on for hours. I made everything—linguini and clams, spaghetti limone, sausage and pepper heros, zeppolis just like back in Brooklyn, dessert pizzas with Nutella. The act of cooking and serving the food I made to my friends was divine to me. I even considered quitting acting to go to cooking school, but that change seemed too frightening at the time. I began bringing six pounds of pasta to work to serve the crew. I had reclaimed the notion that food was a gesture of friendship and love, and it brought me the community I craved. I still had stomach issues, and they were bad at times, but I refused to let them get in the way.

AGAPE MADE A big difference in the way I handled life. When a good audition opportunity arose, I went to the audition not caring about the outcome, for the first time in my life. I simply did the job at hand, not attached to the result, just letting it be. I did the best reading I could, and I went home. I got the job, playing Andrea Belladonna on the show *Samantha Who?* with Christina Applegate and Melissa McCarthy, plus a cast of many other wonderful people! I started my new job, and I loved my cast mates. We spent much of the workday laughing, and that felt good. I was still sleeping through lunch breaks, but it felt okay, and when I got home, I filled the hours with cooking.

The show went on break, I went back to Italy—and my body went haywire again, with excruciating back pain and a swollen abdomen. I went back to the doctor, who suggested maybe I'd contracted another parasite. Really? No way. He sent me to a back specialist, who said nothing was wrong with my muscles, but he did think the nerve endings in my fingers and legs were reacting too slowly. He ran electrical currents through my hands and legs to test them, then gave me a prescription for muscle relaxers and anti-inflammatories, and told me to hang in my closet, or on some scaffolding on the street, to relax my lower back.

Really? This is what passes for advanced medicine? From an expensive Park Avenue doctor? Hang out on the street, on some scaffolding? "Oh, don't mind me, officer, I have a prescription!" Seriously. That's just great, I thought. Just great.

I started the meds he gave me, and they knocked me out. By the end of the evening, I was back in the ER. Between the electric shocks and the drugs, my system was freaking out. I was given an IV and told my liver was inflamed again. Then they sent me home. Somehow, I managed to get back to work the next day.

My sinus infections descended again—and they just kept getting worse. My eyes were so swollen and my skin was so yellow that it was becoming a real problem at work. My wonderful makeup artist on the show and friend, Anne, and I would often commiserate about how horrible it all was. She would pump me up with a lot of pink blush, which always helped me look more alive.

But how long could I go on like this? An actress I knew from a previous job had been fired for looking too old for a part, all due to the dark, puffy circles underneath her eyes and the wrinkles around them. What kind of world was this, where the condition of your eyes supersedes your talent? It's a fate every woman in the business has to face, but it was all too much for me to just forget or brush off as "business as usual." And the fact that such a thing could happen to this wonderful actress scared me. I was tired of it all, and when I got yet another sinus infection, my entire face swelled up and my eyes looked like I hadn't slept in a year. As I stared at my puffy, dark-circled eyes, I didn't look good, but it wasn't about vanity. I felt horrible. When these sinus infections took hold, it felt as though my entire head was in a vice, and I couldn't even think straight. I finally broke down and went back to another medical doctor. When he saw me, he insisted I have a CT scan immediately.

It showed that I had a deviated septum and the bridge of my nose was so small that even slight inflammation would cut off breathing and get infected if not cleared. That sounded reasonable, but what was causing the inflammation in the first place? The doctor didn't have an answer. With an absolute straight face, he said he wanted to drill holes through my eyebrows right near the bridge of my nose to ease the pressure, then correct the deviated septum. I stopped listening after that. This guy was not going to take apart my face in some sort of Frankenstein operation.

Benadryl became my new best friend, and I also discovered that Preparation H could reduce under-eye swelling. I added them to my bag of tricks, but I was only dealing with the symptoms. What the hell was the underlying cause? Then I noticed that my hair was falling out. It was extremely dry and fragile. I assumed it must be from all the styling they were doing to me on the show. The hair girl suggested that the show buy me a wig, but production wouldn't pay for it, so I finally convinced them to cover half, and I paid for the rest myself. It made life easier. I just had to throw on the wig and not have to deal with the handful of straw that my hair had become. In retrospect, it was horrible, but at the time I was too unwell to care.

My hair wasn't the only thing drying up and blowing away. My skin was flaking off in patches, and I was feeling more and more tired. The depression was creeping back in and life seemed impossibly difficult. My ENT recommended a therapist, but I never went. I just didn't have the energy. I went to work, laughed with my friends, slept during lunch, put my wig on, covered my yellow skin and the dark swollen circles under my eyes, hid the scaly peeling as well as I could, then went home at the end of the day to collapse.

One day on set in the middle of shooting a scene, I felt a pop and a bit of pain, and then I felt something in my mouth. I spit in my hand. There was what looked like a piece of bone, or a tooth. I turned to Melissa, who was in the scene with me.

"Did I just lose a tooth?" I held it out for her to see.

She smiled and looked frightened at the same time. She had become a dear friend and knew my health struggles. "I think so," she said. She put her hand on my arm. "Honey, something's really wrong here."

"You think so?!" I practically screamed. I'd had it. I went home that day and was rushed right into a dental surgeon who veneered all my top front teeth in two days so I could go back to shooting. Thank goodness shooting was nearly done because I needed a break in the worst way.

When we finished shooting the season, I hit the bed and stayed there for an entire week. I couldn't move. I was so tired, so unwilling to even try. I could feel yet another sinus infection coming on, the third in one month, and then I noticed a lump on my neck. I was having brain fog that rendered me unable to think clearly about anything. I felt out-of-this-world weird. Nothing made sense. I was also losing my ability to stand. My knees would just give out without any warning.

I was losing my ability to stand. I took myself back to the ENT and he examined the growing lump on my neck. He said he honestly didn't know what it was. He put me on another round of antibiotics and a prescription to see yet another general practitioner, passing me along to someone else. I remember thinking: What for? Truly, what for? I'd been begging and pleading and researching and screaming for help for years on end, and nothing had come of it except a future of baldness and toothlessness and crippling fatigue. Nothing was making sense to me. My fingers probed the lump on my neck. I probably had cancer. It must be cancer, or he would know what it was. Cancer wasn't his area, and he didn't want to tell me. He wanted to send me to someone who could diagnose it and break the news that I was dying.

I didn't care. I had no illusions that this general practitioner would be any different. I made the appointment anyway, mostly because I didn't have the energy to disagree. On the eve of going to the new doctor, I had one of my worst panic attacks ever. The scariest part was that nothing provoked it. I wasn't on a plane, or in a tunnel, or on an elevator, or in a crowd, or doing anything scary at all. I was just sitting on my own couch in my own apartment, watching television, and suddenly, I couldn't breathe. I slid to the floor. I nearly called the ambulance. Thankfully, my assistant was with me and helped me to get back on the sofa. She said I would be all right. I didn't believe her. I was not, and would never be, all right. Nobody had an answer for me. The next doctor would be like all the others. I was probably going to die this way because whatever this was, this insidious thing that plagued me, it was winning. Jackie took me to the doctor the next day. My visit lasted an hour or two, and I was told to expect the results of my blood work after the weekend. I expected nothing, but hoped for everything.

8

my elusive cure

"Honestly, I'm shocked. Your numbers are off the charts. I've never seen this before. I don't really know how you've been walking around like this." The doctor on the other end of the line had just delivered the news: I had celiac disease. I had never heard that word before in my life. After all the doctors I'd gone to, all the books I'd read in hopes of finding an explanation for my health issues, that word had never popped onto my radar. But I didn't care. She had an answer! She had a diagnosis! All I really heard was: *You're not crazy.*

"I knew it! I knew it!" I shouted into the phone, relief washing over me like a wave. I felt vindicated. After years of wondering and feeling like something just wasn't right, maybe it would all finally make sense. At that point, she could have pronounced that I had Bigfoot Syndrome, and I would have been, like, "Yes! I'm psyched! Bigfoot Syndrome!" I didn't even care if it was fatal, I didn't care what it meant, or what I would have to do. All I knew was that I finally had a name for the thing that had plagued me since I was a child.

"But Jennifer, I have to ask you," the doctor said, "Didn't you say you've been seeing a gastroenterologist for a few years?"

"Yes."

"And he never tested you for this?"

"I don't think so." I tried to think back, but no—no one had ever mentioned it.

"Well," she said, switching into matter-of-fact mode, "Before we get into what you need to do, we need to confirm the diagnosis with an endoscopy. This will also show us how much damage the disease has done to you."

"Damage?"

"Yes. I'd like to get your gastroenterologist on the phone," she said.

Within a couple of minutes, the three of us were on a conference call, and after introducing herself, in as polite a manner as she could manage, the doctor asked my gastroenterologist the million dollar question:

"With all due respect, why on earth didn't you ever test her for celiac disease?"

"Oh…" The gastroenterologist was silent for a moment. "You know, I never actually thought of that."

"Okay," she said, in what sounded like disbelief. "Well, in any case, she needs an endoscopy immediately."

The gastroenterologist asked to speak to me privately. After we all hung up the phone, he called me back, and these were his exact words:

"Jennifer, I don't want you to jump to any conclusions. Don't listen to that doctor just yet. You don't want to have celiac disease. It's a real pain in the neck. You have to restrict your eating. So let's not assume anything right now. Let me do the endoscopy. When are you coming back to New York?"

I didn't even take a beat to consider what he said. I didn't *want* to have celiac disease? In my mind, there was no more debate. I was totally on board with the doctor who diagnosed me, and I didn't even consider for a second that she might be wrong. It was like he was speaking to a brick wall. I answered politely: "Uh huh, I see." But the second I got off the phone, I was at the computer, beginning to research celiac disease.

ONCE I HUNG up the phone, my head was still spinning; I was baffled, scared, and excited, too. I had a crumb of insight—my very first crumb!—and I was going to devour it. My assistant, Jackie, helped me research, and we were at it for hours. This was back before there was so much information online about celiac disease (then and now, much of that online information is incorrect), so we didn't find a ton of information, but what we did find was sometimes contradictory. There was one constant, however: The only remedy for celiac disease is a drastic change in diet.

Gluten was out, whatever that was. I also read that I could have no pasta, bread, cookies, cake—pretty much everything I ate on a regular basis. We also discovered that celiac disease was either an autoimmune disease or a digestive disease or an allergy, depending on what web site we found. Some said it was extremely severe and could cause cancer. Others said it was mild and all you had to do was quit eating gluten. I was confused but fascinated by the notion that the treatment for this disease was something I could do entirely on my own. How had I never heard of this before?

My next quest was to find out what the hell gluten was.

I'd recently heard about gluten. My sister had many of the same health problems I did, although her primary issue was anemia. A few weeks earlier, she had been diagnosed with what she called a "gluten allergy," which she said meant that she was allergic to wheat. I didn't really understand the difference or what it meant, and I certainly hadn't guessed it would ever have anything to do with me.

I researched further and started to read and read and read. We found a site that listed everything gluten was in. It was a huge list!

This wasn't just about pasta and bread. This was about pretzels and doughnuts and bagels and Saltine crackers—everything in my bag of tricks to help my stomach was actually harming me! The list also included such far-fetched items as soy sauce and beer and shampoo and ibuprofen, and much, much more! I wasn't sure what all these things had to do with each other, but my assistant and I printed out the whole list so we could post it in the kitchen of my Los Angeles apartment—the list covered my entire refrigerator, up one side and down the other, and then it covered all ten cabinets!

In shock at this point, I was relieved to have more information, and what I read only confirmed to me that I definitely had this thing called celiac disease. The doctor gave me the name, and I was going with it. No matter what else would be required of me, I would do it, and I would go forward with my life as a celiac. For now, until I knew more, I at least knew I had to stop eating gluten, and putting it on my skin, and being in any kind of contact with it. I could at least start there. If that would make me start feeling better, I was ready to go all the way.

By the next day, Jackie and I had filled up ten garbage bags with almost every food item in my cabinets and every beauty product, every shampoo bottle—everything that, according to the list, likely contained gluten. If there was any doubt, I threw it out. I just wanted this new enemy, gluten, out of my home and out of my life.

Next order of business: filling up my kitchen with safe foods. Jackie and I went to Whole Foods and wandered around reading ingredient labels. Over the next four hours, we began to see just how complicated this was going to be. Gluten was hiding everywhere, and there were very few products that clearly stated they were gluten-free. Even Whole Foods began to feel dangerous to me. After four hours, I had very little food in my cart, and only those things I was sure were safe for me to eat.

Meanwhile, whether or not the doctors had agreed on a diagnosis, they both agreed on the necessity of an endoscopy. I decided not to continue to see, or even speak to, the gastroenterologist who had so lightly dismissed my diagnosis, and who had never even thought to test me for this disease. I wanted fresh, clear eyes for this endoscopy, not eyes without an open mind. And I certainly didn't want someone who had any reason, ego or otherwise, to prove I didn't have celiac disease.

I began the hunt for a doctor who might be more experienced, and I heard of one who knew about celiac disease. I was hopeful that I could see him immediately.

I will refer to him as Super Doc, because that's who he was to me in that moment. I was dying to see him.

I got in touch with Super Doc's secretary, and tried to make an appointment to see him. I was shocked to hear that he had a five-month waiting list. I didn't realize this thing called celiac disease was so popular. Once they realized who I was, however, there was an opening and I managed to get an earlier appointment. I would see him in two weeks.

Meanwhile, I spoke with a nutritionist referred to me by a friend of a friend. She was currently writing a book on the subject. She was very busy, but told me that I needed to get off all gluten, that I would definitely need the endoscopy, and that I should probably get on some vitamin D. She was also the only one who ever mentioned to me, "Oh, and you might go through a slight detox." Then she hung up the phone. What? *A slight what?* It was such a small bit of tantalizing information, hinting at so much in store for me, but telling me so little. I was so grateful, but even more confused than before.

Nevertheless, I did everything she said, but the more I thought about my new lifestyle, the more questions I had. After the fourth time I called her to ask her something, I knew she was done with me and my allotted time for asking questions had expired. Fair enough. Next, it was time to tell my family. I wasn't sure what to tell them, exactly, because I didn't know how to explain what this thing called celiac disease really was. I told them I was coming back to New York for tests for a disease I had. I felt optimistic because the last time I'd seen my sister after she quit eating gluten, she'd looked better than I'd seen her in years. If she was looking and feeling so much better after quitting gluten, then maybe I would, too. I'd been off gluten for three days. I eagerly anticipated feeling great. I waited. Surely, "feeling great" would be happening any moment now. Just the way I'd heard, from so many books and shows and websites about celiac disease. Just as everybody else had been telling me.

INSTEAD OF FEELING better, I began to feel worse. A lot worse. I often woke up drenched in a cold sweat. I went through episodes of trembling that I couldn't control, where every inch of my body shook uncontrollably for hours at a time. I felt truly, severely ill. The television show I'd been on had just been cancelled, and I couldn't wait to get back to New York to recover and relax. I thought I might take some time off, and get centered and work on a screenplay I'd started writing just a few months earlier. I had no idea of the road ahead of me, but this was what I was envisioning the day I called my manager, who was also a friend, to tell her I had celiac disease.

As a friend, she was concerned because she knew I'd been sick. She cared and wanted to know the details. But as a manager, it was business as usual. She told me I'd been offered a recurring role on a popular TV show filming in Miami.

"A job? No, I'm sick. I can't do this right now," I said.

"Jennifer, you want this job. It's perfect for you. It's in Miami, so it's close to New York. It's only for a week now, then only every couple of episodes. It's not a big commitment, and we can still look for films for you."

As I tried to listen to her, I felt numb. She wasn't hearing me, and I wasn't well. My mind seemed to be moving through mud or syrup, and my body felt strange and weak. But I was used to struggling through it, so I tried to listen to her. "Really, I don't know if I can do anything right now," I told her. "I need to figure out what I'm dealing with here. But let me think about it a second." She said something about how I couldn't turn this down, how it was just the kind of job I wanted, how I should save up that money. I tried to gather my thoughts. I couldn't seem to get my mind to move. "I don't know. Let me just think about it."

Of course, they needed to know by the end of the day. I was exhausted and I felt like a panic attack was coming on every other minute, but I've never been one to give up a job because of my health. Even with all my health issues, I'd rarely missed a day of work. My manager knew that. She knew that I push through things, so she just assumed it would be the same with this new job. I weighed the pros and cons. I knew I needed a break, but most of all, I finally had some recognition that I actually had a serious health problem, and I wanted to honor that for five seconds before assuming I was "cured" and jumping right back into work.

Then again, as an actor, you always wonder if any job is your last job, if you'll ever work again. Even when you are working, half goes to the government, half goes to the agent, half goes to the publicist, half goes to the manager...everybody gets their cut, and you get what's left. Could I afford to say no? Finally, I called my manager and my agent back and told them no. I couldn't do it. I had to deal with the fact that I was sick, and get well again. But they wouldn't take no for an answer. We argued about it. My manager said I should fight what I felt and not give up a good job. I shouldn't let my health rule me. The job was close to home, and I'd be done in a week. I should suck it up and do it.

Finally, I gave in. I would try. I said yes, but that if I did it, I would need some accommodations. My assistant and I started working on a list to send to my manager. I probably seemed like a prima donna but that wasn't it at all—I now had rules I had to live by. I wasn't trying to be difficult, but I knew what it would take for me to do this. I asked to bring my assistant, and I needed a hotel room with a kitchen because I had to be able to make my own food. I figured if they couldn't give me what I needed, it would be a sign that I shouldn't do the job, but in a few hours, it was all negotiated. I was to leave in two days.

By the end of the night, I was feeling so sick that I went to sleep and woke up in cold, shivering sweat and my head was killing me. I called my agent and my manager. "Guys, I can't do this. You need to cancel," I told them, barely able to hold the phone against my ear.

"You can't cancel," they said. "You have to do it. You absolutely have to do it. It doesn't look good to cancel now that they've agreed on everything you needed."

"Is it good if I go and collapse on the set?" I said. "Wouldn't that be worse?" But they didn't listen, and they knew me. They knew that no matter how I felt, I got through the workday. Yes, that was me, but this time, I wasn't so sure. I was no longer in charge of my body, and I could feel it.

The next morning, against my better judgment, we packed up and went. Maybe Miami would be restorative. I've always loved the sun, but by the time I got there, I'd been a week without gluten, and my skin was so yellow and peeling that I looked terrible. After my first wardrobe fitting, which was a nightmare because my body was so swollen, I went out to the beach to sit quietly and try to chill for a minute before the job really got started the next day. After just a few minutes in the sun, red bumps began to form on my skin. I looked like I was having some sort of allergic reaction. Then I started to feel extremely jittery. I'd been on the verge of a panic attack, but this felt more serious, like something big was coming on. I took more Xanax, then went back to my next wardrobe fitting. It didn't go well. My mood was drastically up and down, and my whole body ached. I was irritable, angry, and scared. The wardrobe people weren't happy with me. Then it was on to makeup, and when I told the makeup person I would be doing my own because I couldn't have anything on my skin with unknown ingredients, she wasn't happy with me, either. I was also dealing with this weird sun rash that was blistering and hurting everywhere my skin had been exposed to the sun.

Finally, Jackie and I went back to the hotel and I tried to get some rest, but not a moment later, the director called me. He wanted me to go out with him and the lead actor to talk about the role. I told him I couldn't go because I couldn't eat anything. That was true, but what I didn't tell them was that I felt like I was on the edge of a nervous breakdown, and I didn't want the director to see it. I could tell I was rubbing everybody the wrong way and nobody knew what I was talking about when I tried to explain why I was acting the way I was acting. I told them I just got diagnosed with something called celiac disease, but nobody knew what that was, and more importantly, nobody cared. In the meantime, Jackie had gone to Whole Foods in Miami and brought back a bunch of gluten-free food so I could finally eat something. By that evening, I was having continuous hot and cold sweats, and by 9:00 p.m., I was having waves of consecutive anxiety attacks. I was eating Xanax like they were Tic Tacs, and they weren't doing anything to help me. I sat down to try to memorize my lines, which usually came easily for me, and I couldn't remember a thing. As much as I went over the lines, my mind wouldn't retain anything. My brain felt so scrambled, I couldn't even focus on the words I was looking at. Finally, I gave up. I had to try to get some relief from what I was feeling. I put myself to bed and prayed for sleep. No such luck. I didn't have to be on set until later the next day, and I was grateful for that because I knew it was going to be a long night.

All night, I was up and down and up again with extreme burning pain and pressure in my chest, like I had swallowed a balloon of fire. I thought I was having a heart attack. I stumbled out onto the fifteenth floor balcony and looked around, and it was like being on Mars. Everything looked strange, as if I'd never seen it before—the ocean, the buildings, the sky, everything was odd. When the anxiety and the chest pain got so bad I couldn't stand it anymore, I called for Jackie. I was physically stuck on the balcony, in a state of pure panic. She took one look at me and said, "We need to get you to the emergency room."

By the time we got there, Jackie was half carrying me because my knees were giving out completely. A doctor coming in at the same time grabbed a wheelchair for me, and they took me into a room immediately because I couldn't stand or even hold myself up in a waiting room chair. My head tossed back and forth like a bobble head—I couldn't control it. The doctor ordered some tests and said I was extremely dehydrated and my blood pressure had dropped dangerously low. (I would later discover that I often react to gluten in this way—yet another symptom that had nothing to do with my stomach.) They gave me an IV and the doctor checked me out more thoroughly. Then, as I waited for the IV to finish, a nurse came into the room and started talking to me.

I tried to answer, but I was shaking so violently that I could barely answer her, my voice coming out in a stu-tu-tu-tutter, as if I were sitting in an ice bath. I couldn't gain composure—I was all tremors and drenched through. Even the sheets were soaked. Finally, I managed to get the words out to the nurse:

"I think I'm detoxing."

She looked at me, surprised. "Are you on drugs?"

"N-n-n-no, I h-have this th-th-thing c-called c-c-celiac d-disease," I stammered.

"What's that?" she said.

"I w-was j-just d-d-diagnosed, s-someone t-t-told m-me th-th-there w-was a d-d-d-detox…"

My blood pressure was frighteningly low and I desperately needed fluids. I lay shivering in the bed, which was soon drenched in sweat. After about an hour, the doctor came in to check on me, and told me that the burning in my chest was most likely from my stomach. He prescribed Prevacid, and said that although he would like to keep me for observation, he saw that I had celiac disease, and they had nothing in the hospital they could feed me. So he sent me away. By this point, Jackie had called my manager, and everyone on set knew what was going on. No one was very happy, least of all me, but I was replaced and able to go home. Jackie took me back to the hotel and started to plan how to get me back to New York. It was exactly what I hadn't wanted to happen.

The next morning, Jackie and I took the train back to New York. A plane was out of the question because the panic attacks were constant. We spent twenty-four excruciating hours on that train, loaded up on Prevacid and Xanax.

This was the sickest I'd ever been. It was my absolute low point with this disease, right after going off gluten. Everyone told me that I would feel fine when I got off gluten, and it simply wasn't true, but nobody told me that I would get so sick *after* going off gluten. Was this the detox the nutritionist mentioned? And more importantly, when would it end? I realized that just because you stop eating gluten doesn't mean you'll suddenly feel great, especially if your celiac disease is severe. When I got back to New York, I was a mess. All my senses were on high alert and everything disturbed me—the sunlight, noise, people, cars, light, even the air hurt when it hit my cheek, even the sunlight made my eyes go wild with burning and my skin flare in rashes. Walking down the street to Whole Foods brought out red angry bumps on every inch of exposed skin. I wore dark sunglasses all the time to minimize the painful stimuli all around me. The only thing that kept me going was knowing it was almost time for my appointment with Super Doc.

9

vindication

He was cold and curt with me, but he could have been the Grinch who stole Christmas for all I cared—he was the expert, so I was ready to hang on his every word. He was Jesus to me. By the time I saw him, I was beyond sick, but he was talking to me in a language I understood. He knew what celiac disease was, and that alone put him ahead of most of the people who had been trying to help me. As I sat there in his office, trembling, mind spinning, spacey, exhausted, and fighting off the panic attacks, silently thanking my diagnosing doctor for prescribing me the Xanax that helped me actually stay seated in that room, I was thrilled to have somebody tell me even more information about celiac disease.

First, he rattled off some statistics. He told me that 1 in 130 people have this disease, and that the average time between symptom onset and diagnosis is ten years. He told me he'd been diagnosing it for years, and that if I did have celiac disease, I would have to be completely off gluten, no exceptions.

He took a brief history, and then he said my teeth failing to come in as a child was the first sign of a problem. He told me all the stomachaches I'd had since I was a child were 99% likely due to celiac disease. He stuck pins in my knees and hands and said I had nerve damage from being undiagnosed for so long, which could explain my constant anxiety and panic attacks. In one twenty-minute examination and a quick look at my blood work sent from my doctor in Los Angeles, he could explain what I'd been trying to understand for the past twenty years. All of those unexplained, seemingly unrelated symptoms were all pointing to this one thing called celiac disease. I tried to take this all in, but it seemed like a weird dream. My sister had come with me and was in the examination room. We looked at each other in shock. I scheduled an endoscopy for two days later.

Two days later, my sister brought me to the hospital and they hooked me up to an IV. This was the moment of truth. I knew I had celiac disease, but I wanted to know it for sure. I didn't know what I would do if he said I didn't have it. As I lay there, I felt so terrible, I could hardly stand it. I felt like a ninety-five-year-old woman, sitting in that chair with the needle in my arm. To keep the panic at bay, I told myself that it was okay because at least I was in a hospital and I was safe there. I would also finally have an answer. I was ready to be rolled in.

As I lay there helplessly, filled with tubes, I started to cry a bit. I just wanted this to end. The nurse explained what would happen. She told me the endoscopy is a biopsy of my small intestine, to look at the villi to see how damaged they were. The villi are like tiny little fingers or hairs inside the intestine whose purpose is to take nutrients from the food you eat and deliver them to the body. In celiac disease, the body attacks the small intestine, and damages or destroys the villi, so they can't absorb nutrients from food. The result is malnutrition, and all the strange symptoms that can spring from that. She said that even though I was eating, my body wasn't getting nutrients out of the food. The state of my villi would determine how much damage I'd suffered and how well my small intestine was able to absorb nutrients.

After the procedure, I woke up to the doctor and my sister in my room.

"You most definitely have celiac disease," the doctor told me. "You are an extreme case. The damage shows you've had this since you were a child. Would you be willing to let me make you part of my current study?" Half awake, I nodded yes. All I felt was relief.

THERE IT WAS, validation and verification. Great. Now, why was I still so sick? I hadn't been eating gluten for almost three weeks at this point, but I kept feeling worse and worse. A few days later, after fighting off my fifth panic attack of the day and putting hydrocortisone cream on my red, bumpy skin, I decided to Google one of the many symptoms I was having. I started with: Red bumps on skin, celiac disease.

Wow! I was amazed by what came up. Not official medical sites, but tons of blogs, chat rooms, and forums filled with other people who were dealing with similar symptoms and asking questions! Tons of questions! I had stumbled upon a whole new world of information and a community of people who all spoke my language! People with celiac disease, talking to each other, sharing their experiences, giving each other advice. I began to hear things that I hadn't heard from any doctor or booklet about celiac that I had read. I was getting answers from people like me who'd been suffering for a long time and had figured out some things.

About the burning skin and sun sensitivity: A lot of people suggested that, in some celiacs, when vitamin D is extremely low, the immune system can get confused and see the vitamin D coming into the body from the sun as an invader. This leads to an immune system attack. This made sense to me because autoimmune diseases put the immune system on high alert. I was already on a vitamin D supplement because the doctor had already told me my vitamin D levels were extremely low, but this really got me thinking about what an autoimmune disease actually is. Although I was still having brain fog and memory issues, for some reason, I was able to create a little space in my brain where I could tuck away all these facts I was learning about celiac disease. I put the vitamin D information in that space. Then I researched why I was still having the burning stomach pain that made me feel like I was suffocating.

Again, this new community that I had wandered into came back with tons of feedback on the subject. It said the inflammation from my gut was swelling up into my chest, making me feel like I couldn't breathe, and also interfering with my digestion. This is why I was getting that panicky, claustrophobic feeling. My doctor had told me I couldn't take Prevacid anymore, but based on ideas from other celiacs, I tried propping myself up at night instead of lying flat, since everything I ate felt like it was just sitting there, undigested. I also learned about the benefits of ginger ale to relieve some of the pressure. I started drinking ginger ale constantly. This wasn't the best idea, in retrospect, but at least it relieved some of the pressure in my chest, so I didn't feel like my chest was going to explode, like a scene from the movie *Alien*.

I was also feeling deeply depressed. Who wouldn't be, I figured? But it helped somewhat to learn that depression is a common symptom of celiac disease. I also got some valuable help from the psychologist that Super Doc recommended I see so that I could work through the emotional impact of having a diagnosis. After my first visit, she gave me a prescription for an antidepressant.

I didn't like this idea at all. I wasn't on any drugs except Xanax for anxiety, and I never really believed the problem was in my brain. I knew I was depressed, but I thought it was because of my circumstances, my past, and my health issues.

At first, I resisted. "Of course, I'm depressed," I protested. "Wouldn't anybody be depressed to know they've had an autoimmune disease for twenty years? Why can't I just be allowed to feel what I feel?" Somebody was always trying to shut me up, and I didn't want to be quiet about this now because I knew what I had, and I wanted to just let my body be. "I've been on too many drugs," I said.

She explained to me something I'd never known before. She said that 90% of serotonin is manufactured in the gut. When the gut is messed up because of a digestive disease, then serotonin production also goes awry.

"You need serotonin right now because the very place that manufactures it is compromised," she said. "By regulating that serotonin production, you will help restore a normal mood, and that's what you need more than anything right now."

Nobody had ever said anything like that to me. I had no idea my gut was actually in charge of my brain. I agreed to take the antidepressant.

I was learning, mostly through those celiac chat rooms, what celiac disease was in general, and also, what celiac disease meant to me. It meant that I could not have gluten. It meant that I had an autoimmune disease. It meant nerve damage. It meant that my gut was inflamed, my digestion was completely fucked. It meant not only could my intestines not absorb nutrients, but their barrier function was compromised and they were letting all kinds of toxins in.

It meant I was in trouble, and it meant that this was my life, for the rest of my life.

THE ONLY TIME I went out was to go to my three or four weekly doctor's appointments, mostly with my psychologist, but also back and forth to Super Doc for testing of one sort or another. Every week, I needed some new test. Super Doc and his team asked me to come in for a bone test, to assure my bones weren't compromised by malnutrition, and my sister joined me on this particular visit to the hospital because she was having major health issues as well. Even though she had been gluten-free now for months, she was still feeling awful and hoped to learn something, anything from Super Doc.

That day, my sister and I got in the Town Car that I used to drive all over town after dealing with traffic, people, and public transportation became way too much for me to handle. There I was in my dark sunglasses and hat, never making eye contact, behind tinted windows. I'm sure people saw me as the stuck-up celebrity. I'm sure they had words for me. I was probably a drunk or a drug addict or a prima donna, or just a bitch. But the truth is, I was suffering, like I'd never suffered before. The sunglasses and hat were to black out a world that had become too intense for me. I couldn't handle seeing, at the most basic level. My nervous system was so strung out and ravaged by this disease that too much stimuli would not only make my eyes hurt deep in their sockets, but bring on those raging panic attacks so that I couldn't leave the house. It was all painful to me: the light of day, the people, the noise, cars, horns, people talking, it was all like nails on a chalkboard to my senses that were on overdrive.

When we arrived, I asked to see the doctor, even though I was only scheduled for a test. I never saw him anymore. I felt like after our initial visit, he had moved on, even though I had so many more questions for him. I wanted to show him the rash on my skin and tell him that the burning wasn't going away, even though I was taking the vitamin D pills he told me to take. I'd been gluten-free for a month at this point, and I was living the life of an invalid. I wanted to ask him why I wasn't feeling better. Why the nonstop panic attacks, even on the four Xanax and one Lexapro I was prescribed to take every single day? His office kept reminding me how busy he was, but I felt left out in the ether with this whole thing. They did the test, and the results came back negative. Thank God my bones were okay, but my nervous system obviously wasn't. I wanted to ask him about this because he was the one who told me that my nervous system had been damaged, and I wanted to know what to do about it. "Can I see him just for a moment?" I asked the nurse again. "I'm really not doing well."

"He's very busy right now," she said. "But we'll set you up with the nutritionist. Come back in three days." She handed me some more pamphlets to read about celiac disease.

I returned in three days and I sat down with the nutritionist, thrilled to be there with her because I thought I was finally going to get some answers to my specific questions. So far, I knew what I couldn't eat, but I was less sure about what I could eat, and I especially wanted to know how I could start getting sufficient nutrition again. I needed to know what foods to eat and what vitamins I should be taking to repair my malnourished body. She sat there across from me in a lazy, almost tired, cranky sort of way, like she was telling me how to, oh, I don't know, fix my split ends.

"Okay," she said, almost with a yawn. "So, you know what gluten is. Don't eat it. No pretzels, pasta, bread. Now, here's a list of places where you can buy gluten-free bread."

She went on like this for a while, telling me things I'd already learned on the first day I was diagnosed.

"Okay," I said. "I got it. No gluten. But what about vitamins? How do I replenish the nutrients I haven't been getting?" I'd told her how I'd been reading up on this and I knew I needed megadoses of vitamins that I had not been absorbing for years.

"Don't believe everything you read," she said. "And I wouldn't advise getting your information from the Internet. But you could take a multivitamin."

"I'm sorry, what?" I said.

"You know, like One-a-Day."

Really? My decades-long malnutrition will be magically reversed if I take One-a-Day? I was dumbstruck.

ON THE DAY I had to transport a bucket of urine, that I was asked to collect over a twenty-four hour period, to Super Doc's office for more testing (nothing about this disease screams dignity, but, at this point, what was a little urine to me?), I had my sunglasses and hat, my bucket, and a couple of Xanax in me for good measure. This time, my father drove me to see Super Doc, and I was not feeling well at all. The panic attacks were coming especially quickly in the last couple of days, wave after wave. I felt like I was suffocating, drowning, having a heart attack, losing my mind, and dying, all at the same time. I could barely see and I could barely communicate, so I knew nobody could possibly understand what was happening to me. Not my father, my mother, my sister, not my closest friends. Super Doc did, though, and even though it meant leaving the safety of my apartment, which I rarely left in those days, I was happy to go and see him.

But I felt different that day than I did on most of the other bad days. As I sat next to my father in the passenger seat of the car, I barely spoke. I tried to keep calm. I popped two more Xanax. I didn't like taking them, but I was feeling like if I didn't do something, I might never make it to the doctor's office. As I trembled and panicked, my father told me to just breathe and relax. He asked me if I'd eaten anything, because isn't that obviously the solution to my problem? I couldn't get into it with him—he was bringing me to the hospital, not something he enjoyed doing. This wasn't his area. He didn't want to deal with my illness, or anything unpleasant, but he was doing it, and I wasn't going to make it worse for him. I rarely ask for help, but that day I needed it.

As we walked into the hospital to drop off my urine, it felt as though my insides were vibrating. I couldn't get in the elevator so I made my father walk the flights up with me. The elevator was too constricting. The halls were constricting, the world was closing in on me. Then I began to jump out of my skin and I couldn't hold it in any longer.

"Dad, something's not right. I'm telling you. Something's very off." I could hear my voice rising with panic.

"Just calm down," he said, looking uncomfortable. "I can't calm down," I said. "I feel like I'm jumping out of my skin. I feel like I'm dying."

"Nothing is killing you," he said. It was all he could do not to roll his eyes. "Let's just go into the office."

"You're not dying. Just try to relax." I think he offered me some gum. I just stared at him.

As we took our seats in the busy and hectic waiting area of the hospital, I took a deep breath and tried to calm down. Super Doc had already ordered me to start taking vitamin D, acidophilus, and, of course, I was taking that One-a-Day that the nutritionist recommended, but I felt like something else crucial was missing. I physically felt something was very off, and, whatever it was, it was making me shake uncontrollably, like my body was in some kind of physical crisis. Was it a nutrient? A vitamin, a mineral, what? I could feel it, like an empty hole in my stomach. My father gave me a sidelong glance.

"Just calm down," he repeated.

"*You* calm down!" I said. "I can't just calm down. Something is wrong!" Then I saw the nurse. I jumped up and went to her.

"I need to see the doctor. Please. I know he's busy, but something isn't right."

"He's booked solid all day and on a different floor," she said.

"I need to see him! Please, just for a second."

The nurse hesitated, then said, "I'll see what I can do." I knew about Super Doc's waiting list. You don't just walk in to have a chat with him. I just wanted to beg him to admit me to the hospital and give me any and every test he could think of so we could find this missing link. MRI, CT scan, colonoscopy, whatever it took. I didn't care what it was; I just knew I needed help. By this point, I was so used to being told that my problems with my health were nothing, that I was done with it. I demanded answers. My instincts were screaming and my body was telling me that something was wrong. I wouldn't hear anything else. My life depended on it. And at that very moment, there he was—Super Doc, walking right past the office and right towards me. Finally! "What's going on, Jennifer?" he said.

I tried my best to gather myself together and speak with some of the knowledge of what I'd learned recently. "Look, I know about malabsorption, and I know something is wrong." I was trembling, but speaking clearly. "My panic attacks are nonstop. I'm jumping out of my skin here." My voice shook as my body trembled. "I'm missing something. I need more blood work or an MRI or something. Please, keep me here for tests. I'm telling you, something isn't right. It's so bad, I just want to jump out the window." He looked at me for a moment.

He patted my arm. "Okay. Go down to the emergency room. I'll call them and tell them to expect you."

"Thank you!" I said, relieved by his calm tone. "Thank you!" He turned on his heel and continued on his busy way.

As my dad and I followed his directions and went down to the ER, we told the attendant my name and that Super Doc had called ahead. They nodded and directed us off to the left, and not to the right, where everyone else seemed to be sitting. I felt some relief—not from my symptoms, but relief that I would be safe now, that I would be looked after in the hospital and the necessary tests would get done and I would finally get some peace. Super Doc was going to make sure I got the help I desperately needed!

I was so overwhelmed that I wasn't paying much attention to my surroundings, but I did notice that it was quieter and calmer than in the main part of the emergency room. That was a welcome change. Everyone working in this area seemed calmer and friendlier. As the kindly nurse led me into a small room, I noticed that everyone in this part of the ER was looking at me. I heard the sound of whispering. Maybe they recognized me from television. Or maybe they were talking about something else, and I was being paranoid. I didn't care what it was, as long as I was getting help. The nurse smiled gently and gave me a gown and told me to change from the waist up. She handed me a Klonopin, to help me calm down, and directed me to a cot to lie down. My dad waited outside.

"Can you turn the light out?" I asked her. "It's too much for me."

"Of course," she said warmly. She turned off the light and shut the door.

I lay there in the dark for awhile, still trembling, but feeling a little calmer. Then the nurse came back in and sat down beside me. "I recognize you from television," she said. I knew it! "Do you want me to put a pseudonym on the information sheet?"

"I guess so," I said. I'd been in the hospital hundreds of times and I'd never been asked that question before, but I thought, okay, fine, why not? She looked at me for a name. "Um…Betty Franklyn," I said, piecing together the names of my two dogs. She wrote it down, then helped me up and took me into another room with a doctor holding a clipboard.

I'd never seen him before. I figured he must be some kind of a specialist. He asked me to take a seat and explain what I was feeling.

I sat down. "I'm jumping out of my skin," I said. I tried to think how to be as clear and honest as possible. "I feel like something is going on, that I'm missing something critical and it's thrown me into a state of emergency. I can't stop shaking." I explained what celiac disease was, and how I was not able to absorb nutrients from food, and that I was sure something essential was dangerously low in my system. I explained that although Super Doc had done blood work last week, I didn't have any results yet. Something must have been missed, or changed, or something. I was still shaking, but at least I felt like someone was actually listening to me. He nodded as he wrote down everything I said on the clipboard. "You see, I've spent many years being disregarded on this subject," I explained. "But you have to believe me when I tell you that I know something is very wrong with me right now, and I can't leave this hospital until someone figures out what it is."

"Why did you want to lie in the dark back there?" he asked.

"It's the stimuli," I explained. "It comes at me from everywhere, and Super Doc said the disease has damaged my nervous system.

Light is severely painful to my eyes. Noises, voices, the sound of people talking, shoes on the linoleum, the beeping of equipment, the scraping of a chair on the floor, it's like an assault. My senses are so heightened that I'm just trying to minimize what's coming in so I can calm down. It's terrifying. It's like one constant endless perpetual panic attack and I can't take it anymore. It makes me feel like I just want to jump out the window."

He handed me the clipboard and told me to sign on the dotted line, and then he said he was going to admit me. I was so relieved! Now the real testing could finally begin. I'd stood my ground, I'd made my case, and they'd listened to me at last.

A nurse came into the room with a wheelchair and said she would take me upstairs. Still trembling and weak, I maneuvered myself into the chair. When she wheeled me out of the room, she motioned for my father to follow us. We went into some kind of restricted zone, down one hallway and then another. Neither my father nor I noticed where we were headed, until the last set of double doors locked behind us and the nurse left us alone.

10

in the psych ward

My father and I sat alone together in what looked like a lunchroom or a cafeteria. I was still in the wheelchair, but as I looked around me, I began to feel a creeping dread. Even though there was overhead lighting and it was daytime, it was still eerily dark here. I could see down the hall—it was lined with bedrooms, each with a caged window. I looked around. There were cages on *every window*. I stared at my father in shock. What was this? Where was I? And, most of all, *why was I here?* I felt like all the blood was draining from my body. I was sent here to get help. Wasn't I? Surely a doctor with so much knowledge on this subject wouldn't blame these physical symptoms on my brain. Would he? My father stared back at me, with no more answers than I had. There must be some mistake.

"Betty Franklyn?" A nurse came over to us and asked again, "Are you Betty Franklyn?"

"No. Well, I mean…yes, but…" I stumbled over my words, anger suddenly overrun by confusion. "I think there's been a mistake. I'm not supposed to be here. We need to leave. We need to leave right now." I got up from my wheelchair and went for the door. Then I remembered that it had locked behind us when we came in.

I was locked in and the truth finally came clear: I was locked in the psych ward.

What? Why? How? After everything, after finally getting a solid physical diagnosis, after submitting to all those tests, this was somehow some sort of mental state? I couldn't believe it. It couldn't be true. I was in the psych ward, and no one was opening the door to let me out.

"Of course," she said. "We'll get to the bottom of this." She put me back in my seat and took my blood pressure, her voice custommade to calm the psychotic. She turned to my father. "You'll have to leave soon," she said, matter-of-factly, as if reporting on the weather. Then she lowered her voice slightly, but certainly not enough that I couldn't hear her, and handed my father a bunch of forms to fill out. "Just some things to look over before going," she said. "If she," her eyes moved in my direction, "becomes out of hand, do we have your permission to use the hand restraints?"

"Excuse me?" I said. "Who are you people?" I felt as if every last milligram of Xanax had evaporated. "You aren't going to need any restraints because I'm not staying here. Call the doctor *right now.*"

She smiled passively at me, and I suddenly had a very clear and complete understanding of the grave danger I was in. My mind scrambled, turning from rage to pure sadness to distrust to bewilderment to sheer panic. Just looking at those caged windows invoked a panic I couldn't explain if I tried. All I knew in that moment was that if I was left here, I would positively never make it back out. Suddenly, I switched into survival mode. I knew I had to put my physical pain aside and blow through the brain fog and start thinking quickly. "You'll have to speak to him personally about that," she said; then, turning to my father, she repeated, "And, sir, you'll have to leave soon." Then she disappeared.

I felt like I'd been knocked backwards into a bottomless pit and I was falling fast. I had to grab on to something, anything, whatever I could catch. The only thing I could see, the only person who could possibly help me here, was my father. I turned to him with every bit of energy, fear, hate, and love I had left inside my body, and I looked him directly in the eye, and I said, "If you leave me here, I will be dead. Please hear this. If you've listened to nothing I've said today, or ever, please, please listen to this. If you ever want to see me again, no matter what happens, do not leave my side."

If I had been there with my mother, a plea like that would have had her throwing a chair through the glass window to get me out. She would have plowed through those nurses and torn down those window cages and we would have been out of there. My father? Not so much. It had all been a chore for him to bring me here and listen to all my problems, but I could see in his eyes that even he was alarmed. He tried his best to calm me down, and himself, and then he told me that he would go find the doctor. "Come back!" I yelled after him as he disappeared down the hall. As I sat alone in that wheelchair in the dimly lit room, I wondered how I wound up starring in *One Flew Over the Cuckoo's Nest* without ever having auditioned for it.

Then people began to wander into the room. It must have been lunchtime. A girl approached me, maybe thirty years old, but with a young face and a blank expression. She sat down next to me, uninvited.

"It'll get better, you know," she said. "It's the same for everyone. It's hard at first, but then it actually gets peaceful here."

I tried not to look at the bandages around her wrists.

"My name's Julia. What's yours?"

I hesitated. "Betty," I said, and immediately regretted lying. "Thanks, but I won't be staying. There's been a mistake. I'm not supposed to be here."

She smiled at me knowingly, then turned to talk to another woman who had just come in. I imagined what she must be thinking—like prison, where everyone is innocent, nobody in the psych ward is supposed to be there. It's always "some mistake." A chill ran down my spine.

I tried to keep my mind oriented towards the practical. I'd arrived at the hospital at 9:00 a.m., and although there were no clocks anywhere I could see (because time becomes irrelevant in the psych ward?), I guessed it was about 1:00 p.m. I absolutely had to get out of here before nightfall. I looked around me, trying not to stare. Everyone looked drawn and tired as they ate. Their voices blended into a murmur, punctuated by the clanking of trays and the ping of spoons as people dropped their dishes into a plastic tub and wandered away.

Then my dad came back into the room with the head nurse.

"Jennifer, the doctor for the ward is the only one who can release you. Your doctor is not in charge here. The ward doctor will be back in an hour. Why don't you eat something and relax?" she said cheerfully.

I wanted to tell her that if one more person told me to relax, I was going to start screaming, but I was keenly aware by now that staying calm and level-headed would be my only ticket out of there. I looked at the food passing by on the plates of the people sitting down at the tables. None of it was gluten-free, or even vaguely resembled food, for that matter. Pigs in a blanket, packaged fruit salad, pudding, something that looked like hamburger, a vegetable soaked in some kind of mystery sauce, cookies, and, of course, bread. I couldn't believe the shit they were feeding these poor, ill people. I shook my head. "I have a celiac disease," I said, trying to keep my voice even. "I require a special diet."

The nurse hesitated. She had no idea what I was talking about. "Well then," she said, "Just wait for the doctor."

I put my head down, trying not to make eye contact with anyone who was gawking at me, probably thinking I was the "new girl." When I looked up for just a moment, I saw a man, maybe thirty-five or forty years old, who looked like he was a million miles away. Our eyes met, and I felt a thrill of fear at his intensity. How was his look so searing, and yet so far away? It seemed like we looked at each other for hours, but it was probably only seconds. Then someone said something down the hall, and he broke our gaze, stood up, and walked out of the room, drifting away again, back to the place his mind had been when he first walked into the room. I wondered why he was here. What was wrong with him? Did he wonder the same thing about me? Then I remembered something I'd read about celiac disease while researching—that celiac can cause dementia over time if left untreated. Did that man start out like me? Did he end up here "by mistake," with nobody to help him? Was he simply too difficult for so-called normal people to deal with? Was he sick, and never diagnosed? How easily I could become like him. I felt a surge of panic. I wanted to hear that he wasn't like me—or maybe that he was, and that I could avoid his fate. Or maybe I wanted to save him. I wished for just a moment that he would come back, so I could talk to him, although I didn't have even the slightest idea what I would say.

Instead, I began to cry silently. Nobody seemed to notice. I cried for that poor faraway man, for the blank-faced girl with the bandaged wrists, for every lost soul in that ward, and for myself. I knew I didn't need to be there, but how many of the others were there "by mistake"? What if they were all unheard, all undiagnosed with something treatable? Those questions still haunt me.

I was snapped out of my trance by a hand on my shoulder. I quickly wiped away my tears, not wanting to look like I was out of control. My father was back, and he said the doctor would be arriving in another hour or so. We would have to wait. We paced, my mind spun, and we waited and waited and waited. Finally, four hours after being wheeled in, the doctor arrived.

"He's here," the nurse said. She pointed to a room with curtains drawn over the big observation window, a feature of every room in the ward. I gathered myself and tried to regain my composure. This was it. I had to prove my sanity. I had to remain calm. I stood up and walked into the curtained room with as much dignity as the paper gown would allow. I was greeted by a stern, annoyed-looking man in his mid-fifties, holding a clipboard and a chart.

"Take a seat," he said, gesturing to a chair across from him. I sat down. "So," he said, feigning interest. "What happened here today?"

Calmly and clearly, I told my story again, from the time I entered the hospital with my bucket of urine to the moment I realized I was in the psych ward. I explained that I had done a lot of research about the disease I had and I believed—no, I *knew*—that there was something, a vitamin or some kind of nutrient, that I was missing, that was making me feel so out of whack, even more so than I would from a regular celiac episode. I needed more tests. However, I emphasized, I absolutely did *not* belong in the psych ward.

As I talked, he studied me, occasionally jotting down some notes. He was judging every last inch of me, and it enraged me, but I kept telling myself to stay calm. After I finished my story, he said nothing. Was this a test? Was he trying to make me crack? I begged my insides to keep cool, even though they were raging. Finally, he cleared his throat.

"You said you wanted to jump out the window. I can't let you go if you believe you are going to hurt yourself."

Oh, for crying out loud! Seriously? It all finally started to make sense. Super Doc and now this doctor thought I wanted to hurt myself. His voice was both accusing and authoritarian. I took another deep breath. Stay calm, Jennifer. Stay calm. "Doctor, I understand that policy, but I'm telling you, it was just an expression. I didn't mean it literally. It's, like, a figure of speech. I do not actually want to throw myself out of the window."

He just looked at me, with that maddeningly condescending expression.

"Look," I continued. "I'm beyond frustrated with my health situation and the fact that nobody seems to be able to help me."

He raised his eyebrows. "You should spend the night here, just so your hostility can subside."

Hostility? *Hostility?* I wanted to leap over the table and destroy him. He had no idea who he was dealing with. I'd grown up in Brooklyn and Staten Island in pretty tough areas. I'd survived my family, abusive boyfriends, even the mob girls. If he wanted hostility, I could show him hostility. But no—I knew my life depended on my staying calm. I took another deep breath.

"I might appear hostile," I said, "but that's only because I'm continually being told something that isn't true. I do not want to kill myself. I want to feel well. I've been struggling with an undiagnosed disease for decades, and I have lost many years due to people not helping me figure out what's wrong. So yes, I have some frustration built up about that." He said nothing. He just looked at me, blankly. "I want to feel better, not kill myself," I added again, just to be completely clear.

He sighed. "Let's call in your father." The nurse stepped out to get my dad, who came into the room looking tired, anxious, and as if he had no inclination whatsoever to participate in this conversation. He'd clearly surpassed his 'good deed of the day' time limit at this point. I could tell from his face that he was done. I was no longer his little girl, holding his hand and picking out jelly doughnuts, but he was my last hope. *Please, dad,* I thought to myself. *Please say the right thing here.*

The doctor asked him to have a seat and asked for his account of the day. Every moment of my experience felt like a violation. I felt like I was on trial, a child, a crazy person, an alien. Call in the next witness! *Thank you, dad!* I thought, as my father told the exact story I had just told.

"Well, here's the problem," the doctor said, talking to my father as if talking to a peer, completely ignoring me. "The doctor that originally signed her into the ER is really the one to make the decision about releasing her, and he's unavailable until tomorrow. So why doesn't she just stay the night here?"

Hello? As if I'm not sitting right here? "I'm not staying here," I interjected.

The doctor looked at me, then looked back at my father. "Is she always this hostile?"

My father laughed and nodded. "Yes. Yes she is."

The doctor smiled, as if sharing a joke about the silly, irrational, crazy woman. By the grace of God, I managed to keep my mouth shut. Finally, my father rallied.

"Listen, she can't stay here," he said. "This really has been a big misunderstanding."

The doctor looked at us both again, then sighed. "All right, but I'm only letting her go under your direct supervision. You'll have to sign a form that says if she does anything to harm herself, it's your responsibility."

"That's fine," my father said. The doctor handed my father a piece of paper, and he signed. I wanted to hug him. Although I wished he'd acted sooner, he'd come through for me in the end. Still, it infuriated me that a thousand words from me had done nothing, while two words from my father was all it took to set me free.

Twenty minutes later, I was discharged from the psych ward. As the nurse came forward with a handful of keys like you see in prisons, and unlocked those formidable double doors, I tried not to look back at the patients who wouldn't be leaving that day. As I walked through those doors towards freedom, I caught a glimpse of the intense, withdrawn man, standing alone in the hallway, staring into nothingness. Part of me wanted to say something, even stay and try to help them all, but most of me wanted to run away. What could I do for them anyway? Maybe I would be able to do something to help them, even indirectly, someday. But, for now, I had to get out, and never look back. I put my head down and got out of that hospital as fast as I could, my father tagging behind.

BY THE TIME we got back in the car, it was 6:00 p.m. I'd been in that hospital for eight hours, five of those in the psych ward. Eight hours that started with so much hope and ended with so much fear, sadness, and just enough ire and determination to get me the hell out of that place. We rode home in silence. My breathing was so quiet, I almost felt like I wasn't breathing at all. I was free from the barred windows and the locked doors. Air never felt like such a gift. I was horrified, and deeply, deeply sad, all the way to my soul. When we arrived back at my apartment, my father took me upstairs.

"It's been a long day," he said. "It's time to rest." He gave me a quick hug, told me he loved me, and left. I felt profoundly alone.

Walking over to the window—that fateful window, to which I'd casually referred, that had landed me in the psych ward—it didn't even occur to me to jump out of it, even though that would have made everything so much easier. I opened it and breathed deeply. The air felt good. I thought about the people who weren't allowed to lean out of a window and breathe the fresh air, or get in a car to go home.

Something felt different. I'd seen the buildings and the skyline from this eighth floor apartment for years, but somehow, tonight, the skyline had changed. The colors had changed. The world had changed.

That sense of security I'd always had, that a phone call to 911 would help in an emergency, or that going to a doctor with my life in my hands would mean he would save me—all that was gone. I felt as if someone had taken the veil away from my eyes and I was seeing things the way they really were for the first time. This disease, my whole life, was in my hands, and my hands only. No one was coming to save me, and even if they did come, would they know how to help? I realized with fright that the answer was probably no. I was going to have to save myself here. I had thought that, with my diagnosis, I'd reached the end of a journey. But this wasn't the end. It was the beginning.

It was all on me. It was a terrifying discovery. Even with all the pain, the weakness, the tremors, I realized I had to wake up, pull myself together, and survive, because, holy shit—I'm really on my own here.

It was like the moment of realization I'd had just a few months before when that 4x4 rammed through the windshield of my car and nobody on the road stopped to help me, but this was magnified a thousand times from that moment. I felt like I'd been dropped in the middle of the jungle, and I had to survive by my wits. I had to stay awake, stay alert, and survive because if I'd been taken unconscious into that psych ward, I probably wouldn't have made it out.

My body and mind were so overwhelmed, and I was still in so much physical pain that I stood at the window for what seemed like hours. I thought, *If I make it through this night and wake up tomorrow, I will do everything to understand this enemy called celiac disease, and if I do make it, I will scream my story from the mountaintops in hopes that no one will ever have to go through what I went through at the hands of this disease.* That purpose in life that I had been seeking had just been thrown over me like a 100-pound tarp. There was no denying that I was not the only one suffering. There were thousands of others out there, suffering, too. My heart broke for all of them and from the injustice of it all.

I looked down at my wrist, at the white band that said, "Betty Franklyn." I tore it off and let it fly out the window, and put myself to bed.

11

finding my way

When I woke up the next morning, I lay in bed for a long time, my head spinning with thoughts. I'd made it through the night. Now what? If I was going to make it through the next night, and the next, and try to get this disease some much-needed attention, I would need to start to learn what to do for myself first.

I felt haunted by that man I shared a moment with in the psych ward. Why was he there? Did he have this disease, but nobody had diagnosed him? Then I thought of my mother, and of my grandmother, with their lives full of mysterious health issues. Could they all be explained by this one word, "celiac," that I had just learned? Super Doc told me, in my first visit with him, that this disease was hereditary. Was this my mother's answer, my grandmother's answer as well? I couldn't believe what I had stumbled upon, and if this was true for me and my family, how many other celiacs were out there, not knowing what they had?

When I finally got out of bed, I still felt sick, still sensitive, still in pain, but I couldn't afford to wallow in it. It was to do something. When you finally figure out that nobody else is driving the vehicle careening down the road, your brain tends to dump everything else in order to survive, so you can fight your way to the driver's seat and grab the wheel. So that's what I would do.

THE FIRST THING on my list was a call to my psychiatrist, the one Super Doc had referred me to. She seemed to be the only one who was giving me real information, and I wanted to let her know what had happened. She was shocked when I told her what I'd gone through the day before, and told me to come in, first thing tomorrow.

"I'll get your blood work from the doctor and have a look myself to see what's really going on," she said.

In the meantime, I couldn't sit still and do nothing, especially since I was still crawling out of my skin and the panic was still coming in waves. I decided to distract myself by investigating more about what exactly was going on with me. I got back online. This time, I particularly noticed how many people were out there, feeling alone, searching for answers. We really were a community, but a broken one. There had to be more ways to bring us together. I began to search for commonalities. I stayed online for hours. I learned how many of those people had been mistakenly diagnosed with mental illness—the extreme version of being told it's "all in your head." I was startled to recognize just how common nervous system dysfunction really was, in a disease that everybody thinks is only about digestion. I thought about what my psychiatrist had said: that 90% of serotonin is manufactured in the gut. It all started to make sense. When the gut goes, the mind suffers. And the range of symptoms I read about that day! Bleeding stomachs. Skin falling off. Hair falling out. People living like hermits, afraid to go out in public because of the pain, the discomfort, and the judgment. The more I read, the more startled I became.

The next day, when I walked into the psychiatrist's office, she was on the phone, demanding my test results. I could tell she was pissed. "Right now!" I heard her say. I waited, and then I heard the fax machine beeping into action. She came out to greet me and asked me to have a seat, waving the papers in her hand like a trophy. "Finally!" she said. "I've been trying to get these since I first got the word about the whole psych ward debacle." She began to flip through the pages, nodding. "Vitamin D levels in the toilet. Yep, yep." She told me this was low and that was low, and then she stopped. At that very moment, her phone was ringing off the hook. She excused herself and answered. It was Super Doc. "Uh-huh. Uh-huh. Okay." She looked at me. Then she hung up the phone.

"What did he say?"

"He said you need to get on L-carnitine immediately, at a very high dose. He said he's been trying to call you, and left word on your answering machine."

"What?! When did he discover this? Why wasn't I told this before?"

The psychiatrist looked grim. "You need to get on this right away," she said. "L-carnitine is crucial for healing nerve damage."

At that moment, my phone buzzed, indicating a message. I listened. It was the doctor. To me, he was no longer "super," just human. He said he was looking at my blood work and I needed to get on an incredibly high dose of L-carnitine immediately. I was stunned. Yes, after all of it, still stunned. Maybe it was a mistake. Maybe it was an oversight. But I wished in that moment (and I still wish) that my doctor would have double-checked my blood work and given me that information before it got to the point where I was jumping out of my skin. I know I said, "jump out the window," and he may have thought I was serious, but it all could have been avoided. I wouldn't have had to endure yet another wrong diagnosis from a doctor, not to mention the scariest day of my life. Within twenty-four hours of starting L-carnitine, I stopped shaking and my panic attacks began to subside. Eventually, I was able to take my sunglasses off when I was outside, and actually experience a little bit of daylight. City noises still bothered me, but not as intensely. I wouldn't say I was functional, but I was more functional than before.

But for the next couple of months, every other day it seemed like I woke up with some new thing wrong with me. Mysterious allergic reactions, emergency room visits, new symptoms all the time. I was in a war and the enemy kept coming up with new strategies to foil me! One day, I woke up and my entire left side was numb. At first, I tried to ignore it, but when the numbness got up to my scalp, I began to panic. I could literally stick a pin in my arm or the side of my face or my head and feel nothing, but my entire left side buzzed with a burning sort of tingling, like when a foot falls asleep. I thought I must be having a stroke or a heart attack. I started to panic, but tried to remain calm, breathing deeply and talking myself down. I called the psychiatrist, since she remained my only medical ally, and she recommended I see a gastroenterologist that she thought could help me.

Dr. Good, I will call him, was a lovely man. His son had celiac disease, so he was patient and thorough with me. He treated me for several months. When I realized that it was becoming more and more difficult to climb the stairs to my new apartment in an old brownstone, he wanted to do another endoscopy. The last one I'd had put me in the ER, so I was reluctant, but I told him that I'd noticed a profound increase in overall pain. I'd always had aches and pains, but four or five months after giving up gluten, it was getting so bad that I only got out of bed to walk my dogs, and they would carry me through the streets. It was like when my mother would hold me when she needed to walk, knowing that if she held me, she wouldn't fall. I knew that if I was walking my dogs—and only if I was walking my dogs—I could do it. But, from knees to thigh muscles to calves and up to hips and lower back, every piece of me screamed in pain.

"An endoscopy will tell us how your villi are healing, and will give us evidence about whether you are also experiencing any food allergies," Dr. Good explained.

"I don't think I can bear another endoscopy," I said. "At least, not at this moment."

"Chances are, it's dairy," he said. "It's very common for people with celiac disease to be intolerant to dairy products. But an endoscopy will help support that."

"Forget the endoscopy," I said. "Let me try this first. I'm officially off dairy."

One week later, all the muscle and joint pain disappeared. I remember thinking, *This can't be! I love cheese! How many more foods are going to be taken away from me!* But having that pain gone was amazing. Every once in awhile, I would test the theory by having some dairy. When I did, I always wound up feeling terrible, but I still wasn't convinced it was all dairy's fault.

During this time, my assistant Jackie, who had helped me out so much in Los Angeles, moved me out of that apartment for good and I relocated permanently and solely in New York. I needed to be home. I sold the apartment I'd bought many years prior and moved into a quiet neighborhood in the West Village with my two dogs. I needed a new space with new energy, but even though I had a positive change of scenery, I barely saw my friends, or anyone for that matter, unless they asked to come by. Instead, I took this time for myself, to reorient and get a grasp on what was happening to me. I spent a lot of time online, researching and learning and talking to other celiacs, and that basically was my life. That, and trying to feel better, of course.

I tried to get out. I tried to do normal things, but then I would get scared about getting stuck somewhere or having a panic attack or getting sick. My sister was still having her own spectrum of health issues, so we decided that we might be able to handle going to a spa together, just to be peaceful, and relax and meditate, and do yoga, and eat right, and just try to heal. We called ahead to let them know that we had to have everything gluten-free from the kitchen. I know they tried, but by the end of the first evening, we both felt ill. Somehow, we got through the night, but by the next day, I was having such aggressive panic attacks and such a severe neuropathy flare that we had to go back home, where I had to visit a nerve doctor.

The doctor looked me over and said, "Well…I don't see anything wrong on the outside, we're going to have to do some tests." I'd been gluten-free for six months and they couldn't understand why I was still having so many problems. I suspected it was because I still wasn't assimilating nutrients. This is more common than they tell you about celiac disease—if you've had enough damage, you won't just immediately start absorbing all the nutrition you need from food the second you stop eating gluten. Five years later, I *still* have issues with nutrient absorption, and my eating habits have become impeccable.

I now knew food was the key, but I was beginning to discover exactly how crucial it was—and how complex. It wasn't just gluten. It was dairy, and I suspected even more. I must have some food allergies, too. The more I researched, the more I found out how common this is with celiac disease. When your immune system is in an elevated and hyperactive state, it can react to all kinds of foods. I needed my immune system to calm down. I had a feeling it wouldn't be easy—but that it would start with food.

I STARTED TO realize navigating this world was not just about eliminating gluten and now dairy. It was also about becoming a detective investigating everything I put in my mouth. Just because something says "gluten free" does not mean it is safe. One night, I ordered a pizza from a popular gluten-free restaurant near where I lived. I was sick for two weeks straight with no reprieve, facedown on the cold bathroom floor with my dogs right next to me. I felt like

I had swallowed liquid cement that had turned to stone all the way down my throat. That "stone" slowly moved through my body for two days, every fiber of my being in pain, every joint, every muscle, every inch of hair. It was like the flu times one hundred. I learned later that the pizza place did not bake their gluten-free pizzas in a separate oven. Added to my list of forbidden foods: anything prepared in a kitchen that cooks anything with gluten. Check.

I was vigilant and pure with what I made myself at home. At first, I was making myself an omelette with spinach and broccoli for breakfast, a salad with carrots and more broccoli, and a piece of salmon for lunch; and for dinner, I would have more vegetables. But then, I was in severe pain all night long. Scary pain in my chest and throat, like a heart attack, or like I was choking. At first I thought I might be having more panic attacks, but then I paid closer attention to the sensation, and it was different. This felt like gut inflammation. I used to sip ginger ale and ginger tea and prop myself up, and that helped. Finally, after researching and paying attention to how I felt, I suspected that I was getting too much roughage. My damaged digestive system couldn't handle all those vegetables, especially the raw ones. It was too much fiber. Nobody ever told me this might be a problem. Also added to my list of forbidden foods: too many raw vegetables. Check.

The list of foods I couldn't eat was getting longer and longer. The list of foods I could eat was getting shorter and shorter.

My sister often called me, crying, asking me questions about the pains she was getting in her chest. "It's your digestion, I know it is!" I told her, and I shared with her what I was doing. "Don't eat so much fiber. Prop yourself up when you sleep." We were developing our own "bag of tricks."

"I felt better when I was eating gluten," my sister said in despair. "Yes, I'd get a stomach- ache, but it wasn't this burning, swollen pain from my throat all the way to my gut. It's like my entire body fights against everything I eat."

"It's a constant fight," I agreed.

Then I began to wonder: if I couldn't even assimilate the nutrients in food, how was I going to absorb the nutrients from a big horse pill of vitamin D or any of the other vitamins I was supposed to be taking? I sought out liquid vitamin D and powdered vitamins, so I could nourish my system more gently and effectively. Added to my forbidden list: vitamins in pill form. Check.

I ALWAYS FELT better when I cooked at home, so I was still trying to figure out what I could and couldn't cook. I longed for the baked goods of my childhood, so I would occasionally flip through gluten-free baking cookbooks. But the ingredients were so strange. Amaranth? Buckwheat flour? Xanthan gum? What the heck is xanthan gum? I never tried any of them because they didn't make sense to me.

Then one day, while I was on the Internet, I saw an ad for a class about gluten-free baking at the Natural Gourmet Institute. Maybe they knew what xanthan gum was. I was nervous to sign up because the class lasted for two full eight-hour days. Could I even get to the class? Get in a taxi? Take the stairs because I couldn't do elevators? I was always afraid of getting stuck, out there in the world, in severe pain or panic. God forbid I would pass out on the street! I would often have these moments where I could not keep my eyes open. I'd be in the middle of speaking with someone, and I would say, "I have to go to sleep now," and pass out cold. Committing to anything for eight hours terrified me.

But I called my sister and convinced her to go with me. I loaded up on my Ativan and made sure I'd taken my Lexapro, and I got ready. My sister called me at the last minute to say she was too sick to go. I thought about staying home, but the more I imagined being able to actually bake, the more I wanted to go. I set out!

The class was in a communal kitchen, and the first thing the teacher told us was that the entire kitchen had been scrubbed down, to be free of gluten. I knew this was important—I'd heard that just 1/8 of a teaspoon of a gluten-containing food can be enough to make someone very sick, and I remembered the pizza incident. She assured us the kitchen was pure, so I relaxed.

It was a wonderful class. We learned all about xanthan gum, which helps baked goods hold together when they don't have gluten to do the job. We learned about alternative flours without gluten, like millet flour and teff flour and amaranth flour and garbanzo flour. We learned about their health benefits and how to use them. And we made all kinds of amazing things—cookies, crackers, quiche! I learned the peculiarities of gluten-free baking, and how to make it work. I remember turning to my baking partner and saying, "I'm going to open a gluten-free bakery!"

She smiled and nodded. I'm sure she didn't believe I would really do it. At that point, I didn't either…but I could dream.

"normal"

With every passing week, even with every setback, I was slowly learning to navigate the world in a new way. I was seeking a new normal, but it felt anything but normal to me. My mother hadn't been wrong all those years ago—people don't want to hear about your illness, and I had some very good friends who drifted away. I tried to be as social as I could, with my low energy level. I would meet a friend for dinner or go to an event for a good cause, but there were always barriers—stark reminders that I was anything but "normal." Either I would eat and get ill, or I would refuse to eat, and then everyone would ask me questions.

I remember one evening, sitting at the table at an event dinner. A gentleman at the table watched me for awhile. Then he said, "So, you're one of those actresses who don't eat? You're all the same."

"Actually, no," I said. "I have celiac disease."

"Oh, wow!" he said. "My wife just got diagnosed with that. For years, I thought she was just so frickin' crazy."

Lovely.

At another social dinner, I tried to speak discreetly to the waitress, but the table of people I was sitting with heard me. They all knew I had celiac disease, but they didn't know what that meant. I remember one woman saying, "Jennifer! She said the chicken is fine! Just take the breading off! It's not such a big deal!"

That made me feel really awful. I tried to explain, but then I realized it wouldn't help. (Funnily enough, I recently heard that that particular person just got diagnosed with celiac disease. She'll soon realize why breading on the chicken *is* a big deal, even if you wipe it off with your napkin.)

Then a friend of mine, whom I've known for twenty years, invited me to her house in the Hamptons. I began to travel out there on the weekends with Frankie Beans and Betty Boop and a bag of gluten-free food in the backseat. It took two or three Xanax and a stern talking-to-myself just to get there. I was still dealing with extreme exhaustion, compounded by the antidepressant, and although the panic attacks were less extreme, they always bubbled just beneath the surface. I spent maybe a month of the summer at my friend's house, going back and forth, and it was enjoyable and relaxing to sit by the beach and have a few laughs with friends.

But it was difficult, too. This particular friend of mine is a great friend to me, but she really doesn't understand celiac disease. She is a "pick yourself up and dust yourself off and move on" kind of person, and that's a wonderful thing for her, but I felt as though she was frustrated with me. She tried to hide it, but I could see it. I couldn't stay up late and drink with everyone. I couldn't join in what they ate. I couldn't go to restaurants. I had to cook my own food. I guess I seemed like a party pooper, and that's how I felt, even though I kept reminding myself that I was just trying to keep myself alive.

I'm sure nobody meant to be cruel, but I was an alien in a strange world. I often made excuses for myself. It got to be that I would say anything to get out of a social event, just so I didn't have to say I was ill. And then, one day, on the beach in the Hamptons, I met a guy.

IT WAS NO time for me to be getting into a relationship. Brian was as lost as I was at that moment in his life, but we began a fast and furious relationship. He was a nice, simple person and he was company for me more than anything else, during a time when I was so, so lonely, sad, and scared in this strange new world. I wasn't able to work during this time, and he wasn't working, either. My money was dwindling, dwindling down...and then I turned around and found out I was pregnant.

I was beyond frightened. We had been together maybe four or five months at this point, and as soon as I took that little boxed test, my first thought was: I can't even get enough nutrients to keep myself healthy. How is this body supposed to nourish a child? I didn't even want to think about the money situation, or the prospect of putting this into a relationship that didn't really seem to have much of a future.

But I've always believed things happen for a reason. I've had to believe this because it was the only way to make sense of the many, many things in my life that didn't make sense. I have faith that the universe knows what it's doing, so I thought that maybe this was my road. Maybe this was a blessing.

But pregnancy was brutal on my body. I felt extremely ill. I made an appointment with the gynecologist and she confirmed the pregnancy with a blood test. They did an ultrasound and showed me a picture of this little tiny spot in my uterus. I sat down with the doctor.

"Look, I have celiac disease. I'm very ill. How am I going to do this?"

"First and foremost," she said, businesslike, "You're going to have to get off the antidepressant and all your anti-anxiety meds."

Um...

"You're not understanding me," I said. "I can barely function even with that stuff. My nervous system is completely shot. There is no possible way I can go without those."

"You'll have to," she said. "They cause birth defects. Take folic acid."

I looked at that ultrasound picture every day, trying to focus on it to get through the hell I was feeling, being off my medication. I'd never been one to want children, particularly. I didn't dislike them, but it just hadn't ever been my goal. Growing up to have a family and children and a white picket fence? That wasn't my ideal. I wanted to be an artist and travel the world and live in Italy. Dogs were great, but a child? The whole idea shocked me to the core, but I kept reminding myself that maybe this was meant to be.

All this happened over Thanksgiving, my absolute favorite holiday. But this was my first Thanksgiving knowing I had celiac disease. There were so many things I couldn't risk eating, and the pregnancy was making me sick as a dog anyway, so I decided to skip it. My sister was making the dinner, but even though she had her own gluten issues, she wanted to make a traditional dinner for her children. I couldn't stand to sit there and see all the food and be there with everyone and not participate, so I stayed home and made a gluten-free version of Thanksgiving dinner for Brian and myself. It was a melancholy day, and I missed having that treasured holiday with my family. When Christmas came, I felt so sick, I spent the whole day in bed. It was the blackest holiday season I'd ever experienced.

After Christmas, I was still barely functioning without my meds, so I decided to get a second opinion about whether I could take something to stabilize me a bit. I went to another doctor, and they did another ultrasound. The doctor came into the room looking concerned.

"I'm sorry to tell you this, but you're not pregnant."

"I'm sorry?" I said.

She explained what had happened in a technical way I didn't totally understand, but the gist of it was that the sack had formed, but there was no fertilized egg inside. Something had gotten started, and then it had stopped.

"This could be due to your celiac disease," she said. "There is a high risk of infertility."

Nobody had ever told me that, either.

When I told Brian what had happened, that ultimately led to the end of our relationship. A few days later, my parents took me to get a D&C at the hospital.

IN THE WAITING room, I filled out all the usual information on the forms: name, previous history, all that stuff. Then I came to a big box that said: Autoimmune Disease. The choices, with check boxes were: multiple sclerosis, lupus, HIV, rheumatoid arthritis, and a bunch of others. The autoimmune disease they didn't have on the list was celiac disease. I asked the nurse for a red marker and I wrote CELIAC DISEASE in big red letters across the whole box. Then I circled it. Then I underlined it, for good measure. You couldn't miss it.

I gave the form to the nurse and we rolled into an archaic-looking operating room. They put me under, and the doctors who do such things did what they had to do.

I woke up later in a recovery area. When I opened my eyes, I saw a middle-aged nurse, maybe fifty years old.

"Can you hear me?" she asked, peering down at me.

"Yes."

"I want you to start some fluids and have some food."

She handed me a tray. On it were saltine crackers, a cup of Jell-o, and a package of juice. I looked at her, and even in my groggy state, I thought about the form I'd filled out, and the big red letters.

"I have celiac disease," I said. "I can't eat this."

She looked right back at me, as if I were some kind of trouble-maker. "You have what?"

I thought maybe, in my post-anesthesia state, I wasn't speaking clearly. I cleared my throat. "I. Have. Celiac. Disease."

"I'm sorry, I don't know what you're saying," she said. "You have what disease?"

Oh, for God's sake. "Celiac disease!" I practically shouted.

She looked at me blankly. "What's that?"

Are you kidding me? I'm in a New York City hospital and they don't know what celiac disease is? I closed my eyes. I didn't have the energy to explain. I shouldn't *have* to explain. I wanted to go to sleep for a week. "I don't want anything, thank you."

"You have to eat," she insisted.

I opened my eyes again. "Ma'am, I told you that I have celiac disease, and you're telling me that you don't know what that is. But I am telling you that it means I absolutely cannot eat the food you are giving me."

She squinted at me. "I've been a nurse for fifty years and I've never heard of that," she said. By her tone, I could tell that what she was really saying was, "You're crazy." I just shook my head. "I'm not going to eat anything. I'll have water," I said. Then I lay there in that bed and cried—for how misunderstood I was, for everything I'd lost, for how alone I felt, even for the child that I never wanted, that apparently never even existed—and that probably never would.

IT BECAME A year of healing on every level. I was still trying desperately to find ways to feel normal, but they were few and far between. One afternoon, I was in the kitchen, making myself a salad and chewing on carrots. Plain carrots. I was disgusted by them, but I was hungry and I wasn't sure what else to eat. I was feeling depressed. If there was ever an appropriate time for comfort food, now was definitely it.

As I crunched on those carrots, I thought about all the foods I'd had to leave behind—foods that had always brought me so much joy. The zeppolis at the Italian street fair in Brooklyn. The sleeves of Oreos I snuck with my father. The pie at Thanksgiving, the cookies at Christmas. The comforting bowls of pasta and breakfast cereal. Even the bagels and Saltine crackers I used to eat to soothe my stomach, before I knew they were the very things making me worse. I missed them all and mourned them all, and everything else I'd lost—friendships and relationships and even my own identity, not to mention just feeling good in my own skin.

Then I looked down at that big bag of carrots, and a thought came to me. I remembered my aunt's carrot cake, so famous and beloved at our family gatherings. I remembered how good it was, how grown-up I'd felt because I loved something that wasn't chocolate, and how much I missed it—the spicy-sweet, moist cake and the cream cheese frosting.

And then I thought about that gluten-free baking class I took, and how much I'd learned. Carrots. Teff flour. Amaranth. Garbanzo. Xanthan gum. Baking, with all of these unknown flours and ingredients. I had always loved to bake, and it was a hobby I missed terribly, but could I actually make a cake from all these unfamiliar things? That day, I decided I'd had enough of plain carrots, so I went to the store to pick up those ingredients and answer that question for myself.

When I got home, my pups were following my every move. "I'm going to do this," I told them, and I started grating carrots. I was going to make a carrot cake and it was going to be delicious and I was going to eat the whole damn thing.

After a few hours of experimenting, and getting flour all over the kitchen, my clothes, and the pups, there it was—a carrot cake. Of sorts.

It wasn't the carrot cake I make now, and it wasn't exactly like my aunt's carrot cake, but it was *a carrot cake*. It was a real carrot cake. When it came out of the oven smelling fragrant and spicy and warm,

I screamed and danced around my kitchen with the pups, like an idiot. I was so happy in that moment that I had found some little bit of normalcy. I wanted some cake, so I baked one. *I baked a cake!* And it wasn't just normalcy. It was control—a tiny piece of control over this absolute, uncontrollable disease that was still kicking my ass. Screw you, celiac disease! I'm having cake!

I had my cake, and I ate it, too. Over the next few days, I ate the entire cake. And I felt normal. And I was thrilled.

And that's when my life started over.

13

ups and downs: my new reality

So there I was, trying to figure out how to live my life. I had my moments of exultation, like the carrot cake moment. And I had my moments of bottoming out, like when I would wake up and realize I wouldn't be getting out of bed that day. My family tried to wrap their heads around my new gluten-free way of life as much as they could. I begged and pleaded and tried my best to educate my mother about why she needed to be gluten-free, but she refused, and to this day, still refuses to be tested for celiac disease. But diagnosis or not, I know she has it. I know it with absolute certainty. Sometimes she tries, but then she says it's just too hard. It kills me to know that she is hurting herself more and more every day, but I've had to make peace with the situation. As for my father, he still says things like, "So, can you have pita bread?" I stopped answering after the 100th time.

My sister's health was spiraling as well, so we could commiserate, but we couldn't really help each other. Even the best doctors couldn't understand why I kept having so many problems, even though I was eating fastidiously gluten-free. It's a very lonely disease. But that carrot cake moment and all of the moments I spent cooking and baking, those were my greatest moments of joy. Besides, going out to dinner was almost always impossible, so if I didn't cook for myself, I wouldn't eat. In the kitchen, I found a little taste of freedom, so I threw myself into the task of learning everything possible about gluten-free baking and cooking.

ONE AFTERNOON, MY sister called me to chat, and told me about something that happened at her son's (my nephew's) school. That day, it had been someone's birthday, and the little kid brought cookies and cupcakes for the class. One little boy in the class had celiac disease, so, of course, he couldn't eat any of the treats. As he sat there watching all the other kids eat cookies and cupcakes, the teacher decided he should be able to eat something too. So she gave him a piece of broccoli.

The story made my sister and me so sad. We knew firsthand how hard it was to live this way, but for a child? So sad. My sister said that child was devastated, and now his mother said he didn't want to go back to school. I couldn't stop thinking about this. That little boy's story broke my heart. So much of my childhood was about food celebrations—I lived for celebrating my birthday with my cousins and a big birthday cake. Christmas was about rainbow cookies and pasta. My childhood was filled with bread and pastry and pizza. What must it be like to be a child and have to miss all of that? I felt so separated from the community, now that I had to live gluten-free. This kid was already feeling that pain and isolation—in grade school.

And there I was, baking cookies and cupcakes in my own kitchen while that poor little kid was sitting in a school holding a piece of broccoli, watching all his friends feast on cupcakes. I wanted to run to that little boy's house with a plate of cookies. And if there was one little boy like that, then I knew there were others—hundreds and thousands of little boys and girls and adults, who had to say no to birthday cake! A simple pleasure that's supposed to celebrate your special day, and it was forbidden? Forever? Dreadful, I thought. There had to be something I could do about this.

My sister called me the next day and told me about a place called Natirar.

Natirar is a farm-to-table restaurant and culinary center on beautiful acreage near where my sister lived in New Jersey. They have a restaurant and often host culinary events because of the lovely farm they have right there onsite.

"What if they let you do a cooking class?," my sister said. I was only a baker-in-training, but I told her I would be happy to share what I'd been learning so far. This was not only a way to educate the community about what it means for food to be truly gluten-free, it was also a way for my sister and me to invite that little boy to enjoy some treats

My sister and I approached them with a proposal. I'd been collecting recipes and inventing recipes, so I had a repertoire. I would give a lecture about celiac disease and then demonstrate gluten-free baking. I wanted to get kids there, and the people who cooked for them, as well as celiacs of any age who longed for baked goods again. I wanted to help people understand 1) what celiac disease is and what it does to you; and 2) show them how to reclaim a little bit of joy in their lives, by baking the treats they thought they could never have again.

I baked up a storm before that class. I made cookies and muffins and cake and pizza. I was most excited to replicate something I'd experienced in Italy, at a restaurant frequented by locals in Montepulciano. This tiny hole-in-the-wall specialized in crostinis and rolled fresh pasta, I had the most incredible meal I'd ever had in my entire life there. They made their own bread, then toasted it into crostinis topped with every fantastic ingredient you can imagine, both savory and sweet. The one I remember most vividly was a fresh ricotta cheese with almonds and local honey. It was the best thing

I'd ever tasted, and I remember thinking, "My God, I've got to learn how to make this!" I couldn't imagine my life ending without ever tasting that again.

I wanted to recreate that meal. I'd been told not to eat dairy, but part of me still didn't really believe I had to give it up, and this seemed like a special enough occasion to indulge in the best possible fresh ricotta. How could that possibly hurt me? But first, I had to get the bread right. I read everything I could about making bread, both gluten-free and "regular," and then I developed my own bread recipe with my own combination of gluten-free flours, and it was delicious.

Next, I went to DiPalo's. I am a big believer that an excellent meal doesn't have to be elaborate or complicated, but it does have to have phenomenal ingredients, so I wanted to get the very best olive oil, the best ricotta, the best honey. I would have gone to the ends of the earth, but fortunately, I didn't have to. DiPalo's is an Italian market in Little Italy with the most amazingly authentic and delicious food, flown in every day from Italy. I also happened to know that they make their own fresh ricotta onsite. I got a vat of that ricotta to bring to the Natirar event, along with the best Italian almonds and honey they had.

At the event, I cooked and lectured and talked to everyone about how to take back your power when you have celiac disease. I told those people everything I knew. I told them exactly how I felt—that all the books out there about celiac disease, all the celebrities on TV talking about it, were all talking about something I didn't recognize. What they said didn't reflect my experience, and I wanted to be the voice of reality, that says: *You have an autoimmune disease, and it's not pretty, but you can rebuild your life in a new way.* That was the real message that nobody was saying. Until now. There is no silver lining. There is no pretty face. It's celiac disease, and you will never get back to your old normal. And no, you won't be magically cured the moment you stop eating gluten. But…

But you can still eat the most amazing crostini, *if* you know how to make it.

A lot of adults in the audience listened and laughed and asked questions, but the little boy my sister had told me about, who was afraid to go back to school, who had been humiliated by that piece of broccoli, he was there. He sat in the front row and he watched me like I was Santa Claus, hanging on every word I said. He was the most astute person in the room. He actually decided to do a report about celiac in order to educate his classmates, and he asked me if I would give him an interview. I was more than happy to oblige. His eyes kept wandering to the spectacular food on the table in front of me that I had made—food that looked just like all the things he wasn't allowed to eat. He looked at me like he couldn't believe what I was saying and doing was really true, like it couldn't possibly apply to him, and yet, it did!

I watched him, too, and we had an unspoken bond. I could see what I represented to him: freedom, normality, and treats. Treats that he could eat safely. When everybody got to try the treats, he ate with such happiness and gratitude that we rigged the raffle for the basket filled with baked goodies so he would win. He took home a bunch of wonderful things, and his mother called the next day to tell us that her son, who hadn't wanted to go to school ever again, woke her up half an hour earlier than usual so she could make him pancakes with my pancake mix before school.

That felt good. I'd really helped someone. I'd made a difference, however small, in someone's life. It was the best feeling in the world—better than being on stage or starring in a movie or winning an Academy Award. It also made this terrible disease make sense to me. I had a purpose.

Food is a primal thing, the most basic instinct. People who can eat whatever they want take this for granted. They eat to live. They enjoy it, and they may or may not overindulge, but they don't appreciate what an amazing privilege it is to be able to open the refrigerator, take something out, prepare it, sit down, and eat it. They can go to a restaurant and find something they like on the menu, and then they can order it and eat it. They can walk down the street, go into a deli, grab something, anything they want, and they can walk down the street munching away. A sandwich. A bowl of noodle soup. A wrap. A burrito. Whatever it is, it doesn't matter. It's no big deal.

When you have celiac disease, that's a heaven you'll never know again. Your life will never be carefree like that again when it comes to food. There is a shadow over the refrigerator, the restaurant, the deli. Every meal has fear in it.

When I went home that day, after the Natirar event, I realized that I needed to get broader with my baking. I had to figure this out. I wanted all the other people who were just like that little boy to have the kind of joyful moment he'd had at Natirar, knowing they can eat something they never thought they could eat again. I *liked* being Santa Claus. I longed to replicate that experience.

That's when I thought seriously, for the first time, about actually opening up a bakery. A purely gluten-free bakery could be a haven for people with celiac disease, where they could go and know they would be safe. I wanted every ingredient to have meaning and purpose and to build health. I wanted to delight *and* nourish. I'd already been doing it in my own kitchen. I could do it on a larger scale.

The next day, I stayed home all day, recovering from the event (which exhausted me) and thinking about this new idea, of opening a bakery. Delight and nourish, delight and nourish. As I dreamed of the possibilities, I realized I was hungry.

Then my mind turned to the remaining half vat of fresh ricotta cheese occupying an entire shelf in my fridge.

I wandered into the kitchen and threw together a delicious gluten-free pizza crust using the recipe I'd developed for the Natirar event. I took it out of the oven, and the smell was heaven. I put it on a big plate, curled up on the couch with the pizza crust and the ricotta, and ate every bite of it, happily.

Sadly, by the next day, I was sicker than sick. I stayed sick for the rest of the week. My body was in agony. I was in the bathroom all day, and I was stiff with joint pain, like someone had taken a bat to my body and beaten me up over and over again. I finally gave in and went back to Dr. Good after three days.

He gave me a look. "What have you been eating?"

I told him about the pizza crust and ricotta cheese. "But I made it myself, and I'm sure it was completely gluten-free. It was pure! It was so delicious, it couldn't possibly hurt me."

"Jennifer," he said, shaking his head. "You simply cannot eat dairy. You're done."

Unfortunately, he was right. I'd tested the theory time and again, and every time, the same result. Dairy absolutely debilitated me. Like so many others with celiac disease, it wasn't just gluten that had to be off my list. I'd had my last hurrah with that fresh ricotta, and that was the end. Dairy and I had to break up, for good.

As I lay in bed that week with my pups, unable to move, I came to an important realization: I wasn't normal. I knew this, theoretically. I'd even included this in my lecture at Natirar. "You have a disease. You aren't normal. You need to find a new normal." How had I not fully realized this on the deepest level, as it applied to me? This time, I was the one who put me flat on my back. I made myself unwell by eating dairy. I had to accept that things had to change, for good

With every joint throbbing, and waves of nausea breaking over me, I came to terms with something: I had an autoimmune disease, and I always would. It was incurable and it was in charge. There would always be more I didn't know, more to contend with, and that was just the nature of things. I knew full well and had known for a long time that I couldn't eat gluten, blah blah blah. But until that day, when I was completely incapacitated by a vat of ricotta, I hadn't actually truly accepted that I was never going back to what I knew before. I realized that, all this time, I'd been waiting for something to change. I'd been waiting to be cured, so I could go back to normal. But there never had been a normal. That was the cruel trick of it all. I'd been waiting to feel like myself again, and that was never going to happen because that old idea I'd been clinging to, of "myself," was never what I thought it was. Normal had to mean acceptance, period. I said it out loud.

"I have an autoimmune disease and there is no cure. So stop trying to live the way you did before. That life is over."

This recognition helped me open the door to facing my new normal so I could move forward. Without acceptance, life just becomes waiting for something that isn't going to come. In an effort to help myself recognize and live this truth, I started a blog to chronicle my experiences with celiac disease, which I'm still writing (find it at www.jennifersway.org). Then I began to work on creating truly pure, truly nutritious gluten-free, dairy-free products I could share.

A NEW ME emerged. I was not only off gluten, but off dairy and also off soy, as I began to pay closer attention to everything I ate and how it made me feel. I looked more closely at those gluten-free options in the grocery store, and I realized they might not be the best idea for me. Loaded with ingredients I didn't want or need, and possibly cross-contaminated, I became even more fastidious about what I ate. No cheating! And then, after six months of extreme illness and six more months trying to figure things out and get back on my feet, I began to feel good.

The first thing I noticed was that I began to level out a bit. I could go up the street without shaking. I would still get anxious, but I could go out and do things. Then I noticed that my body was looking better than it ever had before. I had been telling my doctors I was swollen—not just my stomach, but my legs, arms, and face—

since I was a teenager; now the swelling was subsiding. It was like I shrunk or deflated. The inflammation seemed to be fading away.

Next, I noticed that the puffiness and dark circles under my eyes were subsiding. Many times, doctors told me those dark circles were because of my sinuses, and had nothing to do with my stomach, yet eliminating dairy seemed to fix the problem.

Then my coloring began to change. I've always had this tinge of yellow, and people often said that it was because I was Italian, so I must have "olive skin." Now I saw that this wasn't true. I no longer looked sick and sallow. It wasn't my Italian heritage—it was my sick liver. But now, my skin began to get very pink! I was glowing. I was radiant. I'd never seen my skin this color on myself before. And my hair! It was noticeably different. It had never been so shiny and thick before.

In other words, I looked healthy. Really healthy. I barely recognized myself in the mirror. And I felt better. Not completely better, not "normal," but better than I had in a long time.

14

time for work

It had been a long, hard year, with a lot of expensive medical bills that ate up most of my savings. My new food lifestyle also cost a pretty penny. I needed to start working, and I finally felt like I could actually do it. I got offered a silly job to film a small movie for one week in New Orleans (it was never actually released), and I knew I had to take it, but I was scared. I didn't want a repeat of the Florida fiasco, but I knew I had to do this, not just for financial reasons but also because it was time to continue with my life. I still grappled with panic, but thought maybe I could bring somebody with me who understood and who would help me through. It's always tricky to find food that is safe for me, and I couldn't imagine what I would eat when on location in New Orleans. I needed help. My mother definitely understood the panic, and by this time, she had conquered her fear of flying. She was always ready to go on a trip, so she agreed to go with me.

Each morning, I went to the set, then I went back to the hotel. We'd do our best to make small meals in the hotel room from the one hot plate I brought with me. We made friends with the chef at the hotel where we stayed, and he did his best to serve me things I could eat. My mom and I made the best of this very new, scary situation, and we actually managed to have some fun together. Every day of work was a new battle I had won. It was all baby steps, but at least I was moving forward!

While I was there, I got a call about a new TV show that was going to be shot in New York City called *Blue Bloods*. It was a show about a family of cops living in New York City. Donny Wahlberg played one of the leads, and they wanted me to play the role of his partner. The show had already gone through two other partners in four episodes. My manager sent me the pilot episode to watch, so I could see what the show was all about. I would be the foil while he was at the office, but most of the show looked like it was about his family. I needed the money and the show looked good. It was shot in New York, too. But could I handle it?

I didn't want to set myself back at all, and I knew what a full-time network drama required. My manager confirmed with the casting director that it was a supporting role and not a lead role. After being reassured that it was definitely part time, which was also reflected in what they were paying, and that the show was mostly centered around the family of cops, not around my character, I felt happy to agree to the job. It was a third of what I normally got paid for TV, but it was part time and I wanted to get out there and have a life again.

I was sent for a physical, which is normal when beginning any new project, for insurance reasons. Everyone was informed that I had celiac disease, and the doctor said I was fine to work. It was all coming together.

I was definitely a bit nervous, getting back to my old life with my newfound life partner, celiac disease, but I knew myself, and I knew that if I signed on to this job, I would give everything to make sure I did it, and did it well. It had been a little over a year since I'd acted, so stepping back on a set was scary. Even though I'd been on hundreds of sets before, this time, things felt different. This time, I had a diagnosis, and I knew what I needed to do. I needed to be prepared, take care of myself, and eat and sleep enough. I worried about being able to shop, prepare, and bring enough food for me on set. I worried that my brain fog might keep me from learning my lines. I wondered whether the cast and crew would be welcoming and understanding when I wouldn't be joining them for lunch. But I had accepted who I was and where I was: a celiac on a TV show. I wasn't trying to be the perfect "star" or be the lead in anything. I wasn't trying to look for movie roles. I just wanted to do good work, feel well, and have some fun.

And it was fun. The wardrobe people were nice, and I explained my situation to the makeup artist—that I couldn't have any gluten in my products. She said, no problem, she would get whatever I needed. I was given a dressing room and on the first day, I brought in my gluten-free food. Just as I was starting to unpack it, I heard a knock on the door. I opened it, and there was Donny. I immediately put my food down and went to shake his hand, but he grabbed me and hugged me with a loud and boisterous "What's up, Jen?!"

I was so taken aback, not because of his friendliness, but because I had been so tightly shut down for so long while I was healing that the force of his friendly, funny energy blew me away at first. He reminded me that we had auditioned together years ago for something, and that he always knew we would work together eventually. The bond was immediate and we became fast friends. We had a blast together. I was still extremely cautious with my health, but I was so happy to be working again and surrounded by lovely people. I was enjoying the work so much that I didn't even realize I worked five out of five days for that week, and all five days were long. I got through it, I remembered my lines without the brain fog getting in my way, and I felt a sense of triumph. I could work again! It didn't feel like part time, though. I figured this was just a busy first week and that the schedule would slow down.

I figured wrong. That first season, out of about 120 filming days, Donny worked 100 to 110, I worked over 90, and the rest of the cast worked 40, including those who had signed on for full time. Working built my confidence in myself. I could still be a human. I could still function. It was good for me to get out of the house and be around people and interact and be a professional. I realized how much I'd isolated myself in the past year, even with my occasional attempts to get out and do things. I still wondered why I was contracted (and paid) for part time while I was working full time, and the hours and stress of the situation began to take their toll. I was exhausted, like everyone else towards the end of the season, but I was okay.

This was my life now: get up early to make myself food so I could get through the day because they had no food for me that was gluten-free (an apple here, a bag of potato chips—these weren't about to cut it). Go to work, work all day, sometimes late into the night, come home, pass out, then get up in the morning and do it all over again. Soon, weekends disappeared—I would literally get into bed after work on Friday night, and I would not leave that bed until it was time to get up for work on Monday morning. The only thing I ever did was go out to stock up on the foods I needed, and bake. Even after an exhausting day at work, even if I was hurting, or had worked sometimes close to sixteen-hour days. I would come home, get into the kitchen, and bake for hours. If I could go into that kitchen and make a perfect muffin and eat it, it was as good as meditation to me. My baking skills were getting better and better. I would wake up in the middle of the night with ideas for recipes. It was something to focus on, other than how I was feeling—something that wasn't work, but that was just for me. I loved to bake.

I wasn't dating at the time—that would have meant going out and actually meeting someone, and I didn't have the time or the energy for that. I wasn't seeing the few friends I had left. It was all about work and keeping myself as healthy as possible. It was all I knew, and all I could manage. It was a very tiring year, but I was doing it.

But, as much as I loved it, the pace wasn't sustainable under the circumstances. As the season wore on, it became clear that I was definitely a full-time player, but making part-time money. My managers and my agent went to the producers and laid it out: I was getting a third of what everybody else is getting, I was working my tail off, and we all believed this was part time—something had to give. Either they had to lighten my workload or pay me for the full-time job I was actually doing, so I could get the support I needed—an assistant to help out, someone to food shop, or a cook to help me prep meals, or food on the set that was safe to eat. They pointed out that I had never missed a day of work and had given them all my energy and everything I had. All I needed was to get the support to keep going and doing the job for them.

The producers were great and they understood, but their hands were tied. It was all up to the network and the head producer. The final verdict was: "We'll figure it out next season." This was upsetting to me because I'd been breaking my butt at the expense of my own health to help make a hit show—and yet they put the matter off for another year. The on-set producers, who became friends, said they would help with scheduling for the next year, to make it easier on me.

The second season, they managed to make sure I had at least a day or two off each week. They did their best, but between the long hours, the ADR (the re-recording of lines when there is noise over the original audio), and wardrobe fittings on my days off, it still felt like a full-time job to me. I appreciated their efforts tremendously, but I still felt that the situation had to change permanently. The back and forth with the network stressed me out in a major way because I felt like things were not going to be settled. I was giving them what they needed, so why couldn't we work something out? At the same time, I was having a great time with this group. The crew was great, and so was the cast. The days were long but filled with laughter, and the fact that I was no longer fighting my situation was a huge relief. I wasn't trying for anything bigger and better. I was just *being*, and although the work was exhausting, it was truly fulfilling. I figured I could just continue the way I was going, and wait until next season to cut back the schedule.

HAVING CELIAC DISEASE can feel like a full-time job all by itself. Take going to the market. It's not happening in less than an hour because you have to read every label and look at every single thing you put in your cart, especially when you're new at it. Add a full-time job on a television series and by the end of the second season, I was feeling truly overwhelmed.

I was still gluten-free, dairy-free, and soy-free. I was doing everything I was supposed to do. But I began to get worse. As we neared our hiatus in filming, the exhaustion was catching up to me in a way that I was finding more and more difficult to ignore. Then the yellow tinge returned to my skin, and the dark circles and puffiness around my eyes returned.

My agent and managers could see the physical decline in me, so when the second season ended, they went straight to the network. "Listen," they said, "She's definitely not part-time, this is not what we agreed to, she needs help here, or you need to cut back her schedule or pay her more or something." They said no. No reduced hours, no raise.

What? Why? They had agreed to change things this year, but now, the answer was no.

Over the hiatus, things really took a turn for the worse. I started to get sinus infections again. I had to take prednisone and antibiotics—the worst things for me, but it was the only way to get me through the workday. Then a rash developed all over my body that blistered so severely, it damaged my skin. (I still have scars from it.) Then my hair started to fall out in patches. And then my eyelashes. First, they fell out here and there, and then in clumps, so all I had left were patches of lashes. It was horrific and I was beside myself. How could this be happening? I couldn't understand it. I was doing everything right! I was taking care of myself as well as possible. I was sleeping and eating pure, gluten-free, dairy-free foods. I was cooking for myself and was engaged in life. How could I be having such an extreme relapse? It didn't make sense to me. It was like the ultimate slap in the face, like the universe taunting me: "So, you think you're going to get well now, do you? Take *this!*"

I started asking questions on the forums again, and searching everywhere for answers. Was I somehow "getting glutened" without realizing it, even though I was being so careful? Or was it something else, something completely new? I had accepted that my condition was frustrating, but I still wanted to do whatever I could do to gain some control over this autoimmune disease. Once again, for what seemed like the millionth time, I set out to find an answer. I went to Dr. Good, and he couldn't understand why I wasn't healing. He sent me to a doctor who leaned more towards natural medicine. He was a good doctor who really listened to me, but the fifty pills of herbs and supplements he prescribed for me were not happening. I know myself. I was not going to swallow fifty pills a day. And so I went to another doctor. And another. One thought I might have lupus. People with autoimmune disease are prone to developing another autoimmune condition, but no, the test came back negative. Another thought I had a thyroid problem. That must be why my hair was falling out. I got the test, but that came back negative, too. Ten different doctors in all, desperate to find out what the hell was wrong with me *now,* after doing everything right and trying so hard to live a healthful, careful, gluten-free life.

Then, I found Dr. Fratellone.

DR. FRATELLONE WAS trained as a cardiologist and an integrative physician, and was a celiac himself, so he had a different perspective on health than conventional doctors, and totally understood what celiac disease was all about. Finding him helped me understand my health in a completely new way. He sat with me for an hour, really listening to me in a way no other doctor ever had. Then he explained exactly what was happening to my body, and why I was still feeling sick.

First of all, he told me that my small intestine still hadn't healed, and the damage to the gut had compromised the intestinal lining, punching holes in what was supposed to be impermeable. This is called "leaky gut," and it's a common problem with people who have an autoimmune disease (according to some doctors and researchers, gluten can damage the intestinal lining in all people, even those without an autoimmune disease). Once the intestinal lining is compromised, or "leaking," proteins from food can get into the bloodstream, where they aren't supposed to be. What happens then is that the body freaks out and starts trying to get rid of the "invaders," and allergies to all kinds of formerly benign foods can develop. This, he said, is what was happening to me. He also explained that the stress I was going through at work was taking a major toll on my health. He said I had to respect my body. He was absolutely convinced that stress was playing an enormous part in my failure to heal. He suggested I needed to heed the warnings from my body, take up meditation again, and that I must resolve my situation at work at once. I could not be working that many hours, day after day, without the resources to get the support I needed.

He put me on a special shake specifically to combat inflammation. It contained glutathione and glutamine powder, which he said were crucial for healing the gut and repairing the leaks. Then he explained that even though I was taking a vitamin D supplement in liquid form, I was still deficient. He told me that vitamin D is manufactured in the small intestine, and because mine had sustained so much damage and was still trying to heal, my body wasn't able to make enough or absorb enough. The remaining damage to my small intestine was making it very hard for me to absorb it, so I was still deficient. I'd never heard any of this information before.

Dr. Fratellone set me up to begin intravenous vitamin drips, to get the deficiencies corrected. He also did an allergy test, to determine which foods my body was reacting against by measuring the IGG antibodies in my bloodstream to particular foods, and, sure enough, *every food I was now eating regularly* was causing an allergic reaction—hard-boiled eggs, which I relied on while on set because they were an easy snack. Severe allergy! I still can't touch eggs. Almond milk—I was drinking it every morning since I couldn't have regular milk, putting it in my smoothies. I was now allergic. Avocado, zucchini, chicken, broccoli, bananas, chocolate, watermelon, and chicken, and so on and so on—I had IGG antibodies to all of them in my bloodstream. This is why I was suddenly doing so badly again. The very foods I thought were safe for me had become allergens because gluten had punched holes in my gut. Lovely.

Dr. Fratellone explained that once the inflammation and allergic responses had cooled, I could probably eat at least some of those foods again, but first I had to calm things down. He put me on quercetin supplements, to help calm the allergic response. He said I probably also had developed some toxicity from heavy metals. I was a heavy sushi eater because it was one of the few foods I could eat in a restaurant that didn't contain gluten or dairy, but he told me to stop the sushi for a while, especially tuna, due to the mercury contamination. I had mercury fillings, and he said that in some patients he would recommend having them removed, but in my case, I was in too acute a state. Removing fillings releases some of the mercury gas, and that would be too dangerous for me right now.

Dr. Fratellone explained a whole new eating concept to me: the rotation diet.

The premise behind the rotation diet is to minimize exposure to any one food in sensitive bodies prone to developing allergic reactions. There is only one rule: Never eat any food more than once every four days. For example, if you have eggs for breakfast on a Monday, you don't eat eggs again until Friday. If you have almond milk on a Tuesday, you don't have it again until Friday. This not only gives your body a chance to process each food without getting overloaded, but it will probably force you to introduce more variety into your diet, which usually leads to more nutrients.

He also recommended I get some lymphatic drainage. He set me up with a woman who does acupuncture, lymphatic massage, and other cleansing techniques. She was a kind, caring, nurturing woman with a Caribbean accent, who looked at me with great concern. "You're extremely toxic," she said, gazing into my yellow eyes, fingering my thinning hair, and eyeing my obviously swollen face. She gave me a lymphatic massage, which I absolutely loved. This involves massaging the lymph nodes and manually increasing circulation to the lymphatic system through particular kinds of massage strokes, and it felt great on my swollen body. She also did acupuncture on me, which I found to be extremely painful, but which really seemed to help me feel better afterwards.

As I began this new path—IV vitamin drips, gut-repairing shakes for breakfast, quercetin supplements, the rotation diet, and lymphatic massages—I reconnected over Facebook with a friend of a friend I knew from four years ago. I hadn't dated anyone or been with anyone for nearly three years, from the time my relationship ended after the failed pregnancy. Louis lived in London, but he came to visit me one weekend, and we realized we were both on the heels of some crazy years and were both looking for someone real to spend our lives with. As a new relationship developed, I suddenly felt pressure to pretend everything was okay. I could hear my mother's voice: "Nobody wants to hear your problems." I also knew from past experiences that I needed to be perfect and together and not cause waves in anybody else's life. I told him I had celiac disease, but I left it at that. I didn't fully explain, and I certainly didn't let him see any of my problems.

Knowing about celiac disease and living it are two totally different things. Thankfully, Louis was in London most of the time, so I didn't have to hide the truth unless he was visiting. When we spoke, I always made sure to sound like everything was okay. When he was in town, I usually met him somewhere other than my apartment. I often ate before I met him for dinner, I made sure to get enough sleep, and I determined to be a person who could handle a relationship, not to mention someone that someone else might actually *want* to have a relationship with. He was a lovely, understanding person, but I still didn't want him to know the whole truth. Not yet. Who wants to hear, on the first few dates, "Hey, I really can't go out to dinner ever, and if I do, I can't eat most of what's on the menu, and if I do, I'll probably have to be carried out, or I'll throw up on you, or I'll be bedridden for days. Interested?" Yeah, what a catch I was.

The morning I broke out in a rash all over my body and began to swell like a burn victim, I couldn't hide it. He was coming the next day from London to spend our first weekend together. He was already on the plane. I stared at myself miserably in the bathroom mirror. I looked like a leper. The rash was the worst on my legs. It was disgusting—a prickly rash with white bumps all over it, that honestly looked like chunks of cellulite with skin stretched over it. So attractive.

As if the rash wasn't enough, I could also feel my nervous system taunting me. I was jittery and exhausted. I rushed off to the doctor to get some intravenous vitamins, hoping he could somehow make it all go away by the next day. He told me I was having an allergic reaction to something. He said it could get worse and I should come back tomorrow for another round of IV.

When Louis arrived, thankfully it was winter and it made sense for me to wear sweats. He was exhausted with jetlag, so we both happily passed out early. The next morning, I snuck out of bed, washed my inflamed body, and got dressed in a tent. Just as I was ready to sneak out to the doctor, he woke up and caught me. I made some excuse. "I'm having some kind of allergic reaction to…the body lotion I use. I need to go to the doctor really quickly, but I'll be right back."

But, being the guy he is, he insisted that he come with me. "I came to New York to be with you, and that means every minute."

"Jesus," I thought. "Is this guy for real?" I made light of the whole situation and my "little rash." I told him it would only take a couple of minutes. I was terrified of letting him catch a glimpse of what was really going on—the years of suffering and anxiety and pain. Why would he want to be with somebody like that? When we got to the doctor's office, I left Louis in the waiting room and went in to see Dr. Fratellone. He'd become a friend by this point and he knew that I had started to see someone I was really excited about. When I told him what I was up to, he gave me a look.

"Jennifer. If you really want to go forward with this person, he needs to see the whole package, and part of that package is this disease. It is what it is, and he needs to see that sometimes you get ill."

I knew he was right, but I was afraid. What if he ran away from me? This disease had taken enough away from me. I didn't want it to ruin something so potentially great. I knew he was right, but as he was putting in the IV, he said he was going to call my boyfriend in to see me and talk to me as the vitamins infused my shaky body.

Keep it light, keep it light, I kept saying to myself. But how was I going to keep it light with an IV drip in my arm? When he came into the back area, he was surprised to see me. He asked me what was wrong.

"Oh, you know," I said breezily, "It's because of the celiac disease I told you about. Sometimes it gets me and I have to slow down and these drips give me vitamins that I'm probably not getting. It's really no big deal." I gave him a big smile, just to put a punctuation mark on it.

But he could see I was a bit unnerved. I wasn't a very good actress that day. He asked what was in the IV, and Dr. Fratellone told him it was vitamins. We all chatted and chuckled for a few seconds, and then he said, "So, doc, can I have one, too? If it's all vitamins, wouldn't it be okay for me?"

Dr. Fratellone gave me a sidelong glance as if to say, *told ya so.* "Are you serious?" he said.

"Absolutely," Louis said.

And then he sat there with me with an IV in his arm. We were quiet for a moment because he knew this was more than I had been letting him know, but, kindly, he let the moment be. It was all I could do to stop the tears from flowing. I didn't want to give him even one more reason to run in the other direction, but I was moved beyond belief. With that one gesture, he had done more for me than most people in my life ever had. He passed no judgment. He was just there for me, and it meant more to me than he could ever know. It was exactly what I needed.

AS THE HIATUS from the show was nearing an end and we were about a week away from filming the third season, I was in such bad shape that my managers called a meeting and made the case: The show had benefited from my work. I was giving them everything I had—all my energy, all my time, a full commitment, at a pay rate much less than I have ever taken, and I was paying the price. My health was becoming a problem because of the stress, but I had disclosed my condition from the start, and I had never missed a day of work. Bottom line: I needed help—an assistant, or someone to help with the dogs, or someone to cook for me. Something, anything!

"You can't do this to her," they said. "If you can't give her more money, that's fine. At this point, what we really need is for this job to be part time, the way we believed it was in the first place." All the other cast members except Donny worked two to three days a week, so we knew it was possible. For me, it wasn't about the money. It was more about me honoring my health. I was angry with myself that I wasn't taking better care of myself, but I was spread so thin, I didn't know how else to get through my days. On their schedule, I couldn't do what I needed to do. The argument fell on deaf ears. I was in a contract, and that was that. Unfortunately, my contract didn't say in certain terms that I was part time, even though that's what we were told.

At this point in my life, I was used to my requests for help being ignored, but by this time, I had spent too many years being ignored and disregarded. I'd sat in front of too many doctors who didn't hear me when I told them how ill I was. I worked my butt off for 20 years and I couldn't bear it anymore. The stress of it all exacerbated the situation, and I felt awful. I went back to Dr. Fratellone, and he did some blood work. A week later, as the third season was already underway, the doctor called and said he needed to speak with me. He told me that my liver enzymes were through the roof, and that if I did not heed his warning, then the next thing I would see would be a problem with my kidneys. He demanded that I only work three days a week. He wrote a note stating his findings, and sent it to the powers that be. He told them, "Jennifer cannot keep going like this. She's had a setback and the stress is making it worse. You need to do something because the next step for this girl is chemotherapy drugs. Her body is not healing, and it's so bad that her kidneys will soon be involved. Doctor's order: She cannot work more than two or three days a week until she gets healthier, and these cannot be eighteen-hour days. This reduced schedule is not a joke."

The producers took this information to the network, on my behalf. The response was a suggestion that this was some kind of scheming on my part to get a raise. When my agent and lawyer got on a conference call with everyone, the comment that came back was:

"Well, she doesn't look sick."

Next, they requested my years-old biopsy results, to prove I really did have celiac disease. For me, that was the end. After all I'd done to be forthcoming, they still wanted to doubt me. At this point, people were still questioning me and my disease, as if I was lying. It's one thing if I decide I need to hide my disease from a new boyfriend for awhile because I don't want to burden him. It's quite another thing to tell me that I'm not really ill, or that I was making it up, when it was all out on the table before the job even started. By this time, my celiac disease blog was widely read and very popular. I was always vocal about raising awareness for the disease, and I always brought the gluten-free muffins and other treats I baked at home onto the set for everyone to share. If this was all a lie, it certainly was an elaborate one.

After that, there was a lot of legal nonsense, but while this was going on, I kept showing up for work against doctor's orders. One very warm day, when it was about 85 degrees on the set and I was in a wool suit, one of the producers, who was also a friend of mine, came up to me.

"You don't look good,"

"I'm not good," I said. They had me on a five-day schedule, even though the doctor had specifically told them it had to be no more than two or three. I went home that day feeling dehydrated, exhausted, and awful. The next day, I wasn't scheduled to come in until a little bit later. I had an early morning doctor's appointment to get my IV vitamin drip, and I could tell I was ill. I felt as though I had had gluten somewhere, somehow, although I didn't know where or when and I didn't know for sure. When I do get "glutened," this is the kind of reaction I get. I can't walk, my knees give out, and my blood pressure drops. Louis was visiting that week, and this was the first time he ever saw me this severely ill. I couldn't hide it from him. I hoped it wouldn't scare him away, but I needed help.

He carried me to the car to go to the doctor and get my IV and blood work checked. At Dr. Fratellone's office, my blood pressure and heart rate were both extremely low. He also suspected that somewhere, somehow I had ingested some gluten. He gave me the IV, but looked at me sternly.

"You can't go in to work today," he said. "Your blood pressure is too low."

"I have no choice," I said. I called the driver and told him to pick me up at the doctor's office. He took me straight to the set. I slept in the car the whole way. The driver is also a friend, and when we got there, he woke me up.

"Jen, you don't look good," he said.

"I'm not good," I said. In fact, I could barely talk. I was really bad. I stumbled out of the car and dropped to my knees. Everyone on the set saw it happen. My friend who was my makeup artist got me into her trailer and put me in her seat and put cold rags on my neck and head. I felt like I was going to pass out. I needed water. I tried to get up to get some and nearly fell to the floor again. She caught me and put me back in the seat. I had saltwater spray with me that I used when my blood pressure was low. It gave me a boost. I sprayed it in my mouth, but it didn't seem to help. She called the doctor and he told her I had to get back there immediately. My friend who was the driver picked me up and put me back in the car and took me back to the doctor's office, where I lay there for four or five hours, through seven IVs. That's how much it took to get my blood pressure to go back up into a safe range.

During those seven hours, one of the producers showed up at the doctor's office to see how I was doing. Then she took the doctor aside.

"How long is this going to take?" she said. "We need to get her back to the set."

I understood her reaction—she was just doing her job, but Dr. Fratellone looked at her and said, "She's not going back to the set today. I told you two weeks ago that she couldn't work under these conditions, and you didn't listen to me, and this is what happened."

The next day, they reworked the schedule and I was at home resting. By the following day, I could have gone back to work, but they changed the schedule for the week to avoid any problems. From there, everything started to break down. My lawyer stated that per doctor's order, if I didn't have reduced hours, I couldn't work. We were told that I was under contract and if I didn't work the way they needed me to do the job, then I couldn't work at all. After a few weeks of this back-and-forth, I was finally put on vacation leave, I was told, so they could figure out what to do next. Extended, unpaid leave. In my contract, I was pay or play, which means if they decided not to use me in an episode, they still had to pay me, or they had to let me go, so for those few weeks, we were at a standstill. Contractually, I was supposed to be getting paid. I understood they needed a job done, and that if it wasn't getting done, I had to be let go, but I was not let go for a month and because of that, I was unable, legally, to take any other job.

In my blog, I often write about standing up for yourself with this disease and getting heard by doctors. But what about the rest of the world? I stopped blogging during this time, as I just didn't know what to say about yet another hurdle regarding this disease. I didn't even care about the money, but I thought I couldn't in good conscience let this happen, so I spoke to my lawyer. My lawyer came back and said I didn't have the funds to go up against such a huge organization. He told me that I was just one person, and I wasn't going to make any difference in the situation by trying to sue. He said that it would cost me hundreds of thousands of dollars because they would keep it in court for years, and it wouldn't be worth it. He didn't realize it was not about the money anymore for me, it was about the principle, but I agreed to move on. I didn't need any more stress in my life.

It was clear to me now: I needed to go in an entirely new direction with my life. I needed to take a giant step back and re-assess. That purpose I craved was now sitting in my lap, and I couldn't waste any more of my energy on things that didn't serve that purpose. I decided now was the time to do something—not just sit behind my computer, write on my blog, and research. *Do something.* And, for that, I'm grateful for the situation that unfolded.

15

jennifer's way

*A*fter the whole work debacle, I was spending a lot of time at home during the day, not just taking care of myself, but trying to figure out how to proceed with this huge undertaking. One day, I had the TV on and was watching a popular morning show. They mentioned some new diet book and something about celiac disease. Then they put up a graphic of the word celiac—only it was spelled CILIAC. They spelled it wrong! Obviously, nobody fact-checked the graphic. It wasn't even the British spelling of the word (which is "coeliac"). They went on to talk about a new diet, and how taking gluten out would make you lose weight. They mentioned celiac in terms of taking out the gluten. The irresponsibility about this disease was everywhere! Making this out to be some diet plan was a whole mess on its own, but to spell it wrong? It all felt like a joke. It made this whole disease feel like a *big* joke.

Another time, on the same program, one of the hosts was talking about what she would like to see in a partner. I remember her saying something about not wanting a man who's a finicky eater and all gluten-free and stuff. I don't want my man asking for gluten-free, I want a man who can eat a big steak! Or something like that. It was a really insensitive comment, and after a reaction from the celiac community, she did apologize on the air, which was wonderful. But it dawned on me that people don't see celiac disease as a *real* illness.

These people were all rational, intelligent, successful people, even doctors, but they all had a problem understanding this, and it's very hard to know what to do in the face of that. I have to believe that people just don't fully get how much a comment like that hurts. I'm not picking on anyone in particular because the misinformation is everywhere. It's on talk shows and news shows and the Internet, and it gets passed from person to person like bad gossip. It's been the butt of jokes in the media, from comedians, and even in movies. I get why people say those things—I really do. "Gluten-free" is trendy right now, and everything trendy is a source of ridicule, but the fact is, that for some people, giving up gluten isn't a trend or a fad, and we would love to be able to eat foods containing gluten. But we can't because of what it will do to us. It will cause serious harm and there is nothing funny about that.

When people make those flippant comments, what they don't realize is that comments like that are painful and humiliating, and make us feel worse than we already feel. Imagine some guy who has celiac disease thinking, "I guess no woman will want to go to a restaurant with me. She'll think I'm being pretentious." Or worse yet, "Maybe I don't seem like a man. Maybe I shouldn't ask about the steak, and just eat it however it's prepared. I might get really sick, but at least people won't be annoyed at me."

Sad, but this is how it feels all the time. Even worse, though, it makes others believe that being gluten-free is not a real necessity. Then, waitstaff get flippant about your dietary requests. It seems like every restaurant suddenly has a gluten-free sign without actually knowing how serious they need to be about avoiding cross-contamination. Unmonitored food companies slap "gluten-free" on their product labels without fully realizing what that entails. It's not just about replacing wheat flour with rice flour. It's so much more, but the more this disease is ridiculed and brushed aside in the media, the less seriously everyone takes it, including those who provide the food we need to eat.

The truth is that there are a lot of celiacs out there, and life itself is difficult enough without having to contend with this kind of callous attitude. This makes things worse for the whole celiac community. I don't think anybody is being purposefully cruel or even purposefully dismissive of anyone's health issues. It's just mis-education and misinformation about this disease. I guarantee you that nobody who has celiac disease wants it or chose it or enjoys living this way. We would all give up a lot to have it disappear, yet the mainstream ignorance about it makes life a hundred times worse than it already is.

But as I sat there in my living room, staring with dropped jaw at the television, I realized my first impulse was to get online and go to the celiac forums or write a blog about what I'd just heard. That would raise some awareness, but how was that going to change the situation? I would be preaching to the choir. So instead of posting endlessly online about what's wrong with the world, and why people shouldn't misconstrue and misunderstand celiac disease and the people it afflicts, instead of lamenting how we so often bear the brunt of jokes and are the victims of misinformation, I wondered what I could do that would be more proactive.

I had a ton of knowledge about this disease at this point, but thought, who wants to take medical advice from an actress, and how would I go about it anyway? My blog was called Jennifer's Way to address these exact issues. It's about how I learned to navigate this new world I was living in, in my own way. But I wanted to do even more. I also believe that food is a major reason why we as a community, even as a country, are getting sicker and sicker. I knew I couldn't change the food industry. Instead, what if I could give people an alternative? What if I could create a place where celiacs could go and feel completely free? Free of questions, ridicule, sneers, and, most important, *gluten*? I could take all my recipes, made of the best gluten-free, dairy-free, egg-free, soy-free, organic, allergy-friendly, non-GMO ingredients, and make clean, nutritious products. It was a mouthful and a hell of an undertaking, but I believed it was the way to start my journey.

AT THIS POINT, I had already packaged my gluten-free flour mix and pancake mix, and was making them available on my blog, but it wasn't enough. The interaction with others through my blog was great, but I wanted to do more.

I think the universe points you in the direction you need to go, and this was my direction. I was standing in the middle of my apartment feeling so frustrated with what I saw on that television. That's when I thought, "No. I'm not going to do that. I'm going to be a part of the solution." Even if I just made a small step, it would be a step in the right direction. I would open my bakery.

But if I was really going to open a bakery, I needed money. I began talking to some people about the idea, and I had a lot of meetings. I discovered one investor was going down some not-so-appropriate avenues and using my name. One memorable meeting with someone very high up in the food industry was a disaster. He looked me in the eye and said, "Jennifer, let's be real. This bakery and this product aren't exactly a necessity. Nobody is going to come into your bakery just to get a gluten-free cupcake."

"You are absolutely wrong," I said. "*Absolutely wrong.*"

Everyone told me not to do it. Even my family. My mom said, "Jen, you don't know what you're getting into. Opening up your own business is a lot of work. Can't you just sell your idea and sit back and collect the checks and rest?" My family had some concern because of my health. They wanted me to take an easier road. But I've never had an easy road. I figured, why the hell start now?

So I went into my own bank account, to see if I could start this bakery without any help. I came up short. And then, one afternoon, as I sat there crying after a particularly cruel meeting during which I was told I should really just go sell my recipes to the health and beauty community as a diet and call it a day, Louis came up behind me and put his arms around me.

"I'll give you the rest of the money," he said. "I believe in you and I believe in your products and I see what you deal with, and I know we can do this." He could have closed his eyes and supported me with words only, but he didn't. He put his money where his heart was.

I found a spot on the block where I had always dreamt my bakery would be, in a former hair salon that had graffiti all over the walls and sheetrock covering beautiful old brick. We wanted the place to feel like a cozy home and a peaceful retreat. It's a very healthy block in the East Village in New York City, with a raw restaurant across the way, a juice press serving fresh juices a few doors down, a raw vitamin store, even a famous Russian bathhouse that has steam, sauna, and massage. It's just one storefront after another offering the healthiest things out there. It is the perfect spot for me.

So, without listening to the many friends in the restaurant business who told me not to do it, without listening to my family who told me not to do it, without listening to all the friends and acquaintances and colleagues who told me not to do it, I did it anyway.

And boy, were they all right!

I say that with a laugh, but it has been extremely difficult, even to get the place open, because of all the regulations and rules a new business must comply with in New York City. After running through three contractors, Louis and I soon realized we would have to do most of the work ourselves. We tore out the sheetrock to expose the brick. We added beams and antiques and even made a counter out of an old antique door (it still has the locks and hardware on it). When our final contractor kept extending the deadlines, Louis and I fired that company, then got in there with sanders and finished off all the wood ourselves.

We put white subway tile across half of one wall, and then we added a big chalkboard. The bakery is about relearning how to live and experience food, and the chalkboard is a reminder of that. We change what's on there, from specials to facts about celiac disease or gluten. Right now, for example, it says, "Did you know many prescription medications contain gluten?"

I turned old potato sacks from a flea market into cushions for the chairs. The big communal table came from an antique market, and the bakery cases came from Etsy.com. We painted the bathroom and hung posters, and it was all truly a labor of love. Today, it is just the cozy, peaceful retreat I imagined, but it was quite a job getting there—the health department codes, the handicapped accessibility requirements, the ten-foot turnaround, the proper sinks, the six-foot turnaround, the food protection certificate. I had to go to Harlem and take the test with all the other wannabe waiters and shop owners and bartenders. It was a drastic change from working on a TV set, just wild. We know so much more now than when we started, and it's certainly not glamorous. I spend my days covered in flour, washing dishes, mopping the floor. But it's my bakery. I wanted it to feel like walking into your grandma's kitchen and feeling safe, and just relaxing and enjoying the food, and I think it does feel exactly like that. I might not have done everything right, or in the most efficient or practical way, but I did it.

WHEN PEOPLE COME into the bakery, the first thing they notice is the smell—it doesn't smell like a "specialty bakery"—it smells like fresh bread and cookies, like cinnamon and vanilla. Every day when I walk in, that smell hits me in the face and takes me back to that happy, warm, welcoming time in my childhood when food was exciting and comforting and represented everything good.

When we're baking the chocolate chip cookies, the smell takes me back to the days when I baked cookies with my sister at Christmas. When we're baking the onion bagels, the whole shop smells like savory onions and soft bread, and people marvel at the chewy texture. The pumpkin muffins fill the bakery with the scent of cinnamon and nutmeg. And the bread! Just like I remembered. It's not easy to get that airy texture in bread. So much gluten-free bread is like dense clay. Or to get that little bit of crunch on the outside of the cookie, but the soft center. I never stop experimenting. It's a science and an art, and the bakery is my laboratory and my studio. All I have to do is go into the bakery, and I can forget everything else and focus on nothing but what I am creating. It has always been and remains my very favorite thing to do.

Now, every day, people come in to my bakery and get to eat something *safely*. This is the other huge part of the bakery for me. That refuge I wanted for myself has also become a refuge for everyone who walks in the door. It's a strange thing that happens when people see me. I think that if they have heard I own the bakery, they don't really expect that I'll be behind the counter. I can't count the number of times that someone is standing there talking to the girl at the register, and I walk out from the back in my flour-covered apron, and the customer sees me and just stops talking, and stands there, and then bursts into tears. I guarantee it's not because they loved what I did in TV show number ten. It's more about coming face-to-face with somebody who gets it, really gets it. Gets what it truly means to have this disease. On many occasions, it has brought people to tears. This means everything to someone who deals with such difficulty every day, especially when their families don't get it, their parents and siblings don't get it, their colleagues, their bosses, their doctors don't get it. People tell me they have been suffering alone, and trying so hard *not* to suffer, or, at least, not to make anyone else suffer. This disease wreaks havoc on every aspect of your life.

I understand, and in the everyday life of a celiac, the people who truly understand are few and far between. I think people have a few basic needs. They want love, they want to feel safe, and they want to be heard. Celiac disease takes away two of those things. You are not heard. The average time for diagnosis is eight to ten years. And you do not feel safe anymore, in any situation where food is involved. For me, who was so enraptured by food, who had such a love affair with food, who loved to travel independently and try new foods and experience new things and immerse myself in new cultures, celiac disease took all that away. As far as feeling loved, it can be hard when you don't have a partner who understands. Family friends and personal relationships all get tested when you make such a drastic change in your life. When people come into the bakery, it's like they let out a huge sigh of relief. Sometimes, they even apologize for crying. That's the one thing I hear from people with celiac all the time. They are always apologizing. They are sorry for being an inconvenience, sorry for being annoying, sorry for not being any fun, sorry for being so much of a "problem." You have to get to the point where you forgive yourself for having celiac disease—for having *any* disease. And eventually, you also have to get to the point where you forgive the people around you who don't understand, if you want any peace. They can't possibly understand what you're going through. It's not their fault, either.

This is why it's so crucial for us to find support, and that right there is one of the main reasons why I opened this bakery—not only to provide a place where I can give people back a feeling of safety and joy when they eat, but to create an environment where everyone gets it, where you don't have to make any excuses, where you never have to apologize. Where you don't even have to say a word. Or you can share your story. Or you can simply order a cupcake, without discussion, without questions. You can just order a cupcake, and eat it, and enjoy it, and feel happy.

So, as hard as the bakery has been, every square inch of reclaimed wood and bakery case glass, every tablespoon of gluten-free flour, every baking sheet and platter and chair and piece of chalk in that bakery came out of a labor of the greatest love. There are times when I still think, "What the hell did I do, opening this place?" Yet, it's as rewarding as anything I have ever done, a million times over. No movie can compare. No award can compare. Nothing can compare to being able to deal with people on this level and make them feel like they're not crazy. Like they are heard. Because, in this bakery, they are.

two

Your Journey

16

what exactly is celiac disease?

*S*o, what does all this mean? Where do we go from here? You've heard my story up to this point, and I've shared my life with you in the hope that I can show by example the twists and turns of this disease. Maybe you will recognize parts of your story in parts of my story—or in the stories of some of the people who've come to my bakery. Maybe this will help you cope, or not feel so alone. Or maybe this will give you a light bulb moment and you will realize that you might actually have celiac disease, too.

Now it's time to talk about you.

If you've just been diagnosed, you might be scared, or confused, or just hungry for information. (Or just plain *hungry!*) If you haven't been diagnosed yet, you might be wondering if you should get to your doctor, but afraid that he might not hear you or diagnose you properly. I hear that! In this second half of the book, I want to tell you what I've learned—about celiac disease, about gluten, and about everything your doctor probably won't or didn't tell you. This will help you make the right decisions for yourself and take charge of your life again—because nobody else is going to do it for you.

This is the book I wish I'd had when I was first diagnosed, when I knew nothing and nobody was there to help and guide me. I wish someone would have sat down with me to say, "Here's what's going to happen now," and "Here's what you need to do," and "Here's what to watch out for," and "Here's what you can eat when you feel like the whole world is poison to you."

In that spirit, I'll tell you all about celiac disease, and what you should know, and then I'll give you some ideas, based on my own treatment and what's worked for me. Everything I tell you that I did is, of course, "Jennifer's Way," and it might not be your way, but then again, a lot of what I tell you might work for you. I just want to give you options and ideas for what you can do to start feeling better and regaining control over your life. It takes a village of celiacs to help anyone learn how to thrive with this illness, so here I am, ready to lead the way. Let's start by talking about exactly what you're dealing with here.

Just What the Hell Is Celiac Disease?

When I first got my diagnosis, I was so relieved to know I had something real and it wasn't all in my head. Great. But my very next question was, "What the hell is celiac disease?" So let's clear this up right now. In case you haven't already researched the heck out of your diagnosis, here are some basics that I learned:

Celiac disease is a very common autoimmune disease, which means that for some unknown reason (probably part genetics, part immunological, and part environmental), your immune system gets confused by gluten, thinking it is some dangerous foreign invader like bacteria or a virus. It was once thought to be a rare intestinal childhood disorder, but now, as you know, it is a common condition with a wide spectrum of manifestations. (Some people still operate under the false assumption that it is rare.)

Celiac disease causes the production of antibodies to the gluten protein, which then begin attacking your small intestine. The villi, which are the microscopic protuberances along the inner wall of your small intestine covered with tiny hairs that absorb nutrients from food, get slaughtered during this immune system assault. These villi are responsible for making (or manufacturing) vitamin D3, as well as the important brain hormone or neurotransmitter called se-rotonin. This is why there are so many brain and nerve problems associated with celiac disease (like depression, anxiety, memory loss, "brain fog," and insomnia). Most of the serotonin in your body is made in the small intestine, not the brain.

Over the course of years, they can become completely flattened and damaged so that they can't absorb nutrients. That means you eat food, but you don't absorb the nutrients. Your body becomes malnourished, like you are on a desert island, slowly starving. To survive, your body begins taking nutrients where it can—first from your bones, then from your nervous system (where it attacked me), and from wherever else it can easily extract them. That leads to a laundry list of health problems related to malnutrition that will manifest differently for each person. In some, the symptoms are ob-vious. In others, they are subtle. Some people have gastrointestinal symptoms. Some have nervous system symptoms. Some have no obvious symptoms, yet the damage is being done. Sometimes, the effects wait insidiously, then go off like a bomb as soon as you expe-rience stress or trauma. I have learned that these features that have nothing to do with your intestines (called "extra-intestinal features") range from anemia to osteoporosis to cancer, as well as to other au-toimmune diseases, especially those affecting the thyroid.

There are different theories about why some people get celiac disease and others don't. Some of it is genetic, but some kind of stressor probably sets it off. This could be physical stress, like a virus or a bacterial infection in childhood, or emotional stress, like an ex-tremely stressful event—an accident, a death in the family, or the chronic stress of a difficult life. A recent report from the Institute for Responsible Technology in Fairfield, Iowa, has proposed a link between genetically modified food and gluten-related disorders in some people. So much of the food we eat is far from its natural state, and that might confuse our bodies into launching an immune attack on itself.

But why is gluten the target? Of all the proteins in all the world, what is the big problem with this one, and why does about 1 to 3% of the population react so violently against it? (If you have a parent, sibling, or child with celiac disease, your risk goes up to about 1 in 22.) Gluten is a protein that naturally occurs in wheat, barley, rye, and other similar grains. (It does *not* occur in plain rice, corn, potatoes, quinoa, amaranth, teff, millet, or buckwheat.) Gluten is rich in glutamine and proline, and poorly absorbed in the human upper digestive tract, even in people who don't have celiac disease. It also contains gliadin. Gliadin is the alcohol fraction of gluten, and it is soluble. Gliadin is the reason for much of the toxicity associated with gluten. This is very important because undigested gliadin is resistant to the breakdown from the stomach, pancreas, and those tiny hairs on the villi in the small intestine. As you can see, gluten is a tough sell for *anybody's* digestion. It's just a particularly dangerous problem in people with celiac disease.

But it's in almost everything most people eat. In food, gluten is like a glue that holds things together. When you knead bread until it gets those elastic strings, that's gluten. When bread rises, the gluten forms little pillows of gas. Without gluten or something that does a similar thing, baked goods crumble and fall apart. This all sounds fine, right?

But wheat has changed a lot in the thousands of years since people first started eating it. It's been selectively bred to be heartier and more resistant, and it's become more resistant to digestion in the process. We don't know for sure whether it is the changes in wheat that have led to an increased incidence of celiac disease in this century, or whether it is simply because we eat so much more of it than we used to. Or maybe it is something else—our immune systems have been broken down by a chemically polluted environment, or something else is causing our immunity to go awry. There is a theory that getting a virus as a child can trigger autoimmune disease in genetically susceptible people because the gluten protein resembles certain viruses, so in fighting the virus, the body gets confused and starts attacking gluten, and therefore, your body. In any case, scientists believe the increased rate of celiac disease is *not* just due to higher rates of diagnosis. Something else is going on. Our bodies are objecting to gluten, for whatever reason. Even if you never know the reason, if you have celiac disease, you absolutely have to get gluten out of your life.

Celiac Symptoms

People often ask me my symptoms, and I hesitate to name them because I don't want anyone to think that if he or she has different symptoms, then celiac disease isn't to blame. The truth is that celiac disease manifests itself in a huge variety of symptoms. You might have stomach problems, or only neurological symptoms like anxiety and depression, or you might have bone and dental defects, or infertility, or any number of other symptoms. You might have many mild symptoms, or just one very serious one. Or you might think you have no symptoms at all (although once you know you have celiac disease, you may find that when you look back, you see the symptoms you didn't realize could have been related, but probably were).

Everybody who has celiac disease experiences it in a different way because genetics and your individual makeup determine how the disease, not to mention the resulting malnutrition, will affect you. So please don't think that if you don't have a symptom, I'm not talking about you. I'm talking about *all of you.*

With that understanding, here are some of the symptoms, although this is not a complete list. You won't have all of these symptoms, and you may not think you have any of them. Or you may have symptoms that aren't on this list. I have divided this by symptom type:

GASTROINTESTINAL SYMPTOMS

This is the most common symptom category. Many people with celiac disease are first misdiagnosed with other gastrointestinal issues like irritable bowel syndrome (IBS), inflammatory bowel disease (IBD), or Crohn's disease. Other diseases sometimes confused with celiac disease (because they also destroy the intestinal villi) are tropical sprue, intestinal lymphoma, eosinophilic gastroenteritis, and Whipple's Disease. I mention these not to scare you, but to show you that there are other diseases similar to celiac disease that are *not* celiac disease.

But remember, gastrointestinal symptoms do not happen to everyone. In fact, up to half or even more people with celiac disease may experience *no discernible gastrointestinal symptoms.* Many, many people have completely different symptoms.

Think of symptoms as either gastrointestinal, or extra-intestinal. Those with classic or symptomatic gastrointestinal complaints vary, but here is a list of some of the typical symptoms:

Chronic diarrhea
Severe constipation
Abdominal bloating
Abdominal pain
Weakness
Malabsorption
Vomiting
Burning stomach/inflammation
Nausea
Anemia

Weight loss

Failure to thrive in children

Malabsorption is particularly important because it can cause so many other symptoms, so let's take a minute to define it. Malabsorption literally means "bad absorption." It can cause weight loss, failure to thrive in children, gas, and, most importantly, a variety of vitamin and mineral deficiencies.

The most common extra-intestinal symptom is anemia. This happens because of the lack of iron absorption, but it can also be caused by a B12 deficiency. This is why I frequently need either a B12 injection or an intravenous drip of minerals and vitamins. I want you to understand that this has been real for me, and, for a long time, it has been hellish.

NERVOUS SYSTEM SYMPTOMS

For me, the neurologic (nervous system) symptoms have by far been the worst. The most common neurologic symptom in people with celiac disease is neuropathy (nerve pain), which I suffer from. Another is dementia, which I do not have, but it happens to some people. Also, both anxiety and depression are linked to celiac disease. Here are some of the common nervous system symptoms:

Brain fog

Depression

Anxiety

Panic attacks

Neuropathy (numbness and weakness in nerves)

Ataxia (uncoordinated, jerky movements)

Palsy (especially weakness and drooping of facial
    muscles)

Various studies also offer evidence that other mental health issues could be related to the ravages of celiac disease, like:

Schizophrenia
Autism
Bipolar disorder
Attention deficit hyperactivity disorder (ADHD)
Psychosis
Dementia

OTHER SYMPTOMS

There are a host of other symptoms that seem completely unrelated to your small intestine or nervous system, but are directly related to nutritional deficiencies. I've experienced many of these. Maybe you'll recognize some yourself. They include:

1. Liver symptoms. The elevation of my liver enzymes stumped many doctors, but this is commonly associated with celiac disease. I know now that 10% of all patients with unexplained liver enzyme elevation have celiac disease.

2. Bone disorders. Osteopenia and osteoporosis are commonly seen in patients with celiac disease. I never understood this, but now it makes sense to me. If the body is inflamed, which also means acidic, then it has to get balanced and become more alkaline. A major source of minerals that promote alkalinity exist in the bones, so the body leaches calcium to balance itself. It's a survival mechanism. There are studies that have evaluated bone mineral density in celiac patients. The good news is that a truly gluten-free diet can reverse bone loss, so if you have this problem, you can repair your bones with diet until they are comparable to someone without celiac disease.

3. Other autoimmune diseases. You would think if you have one, you won't have to suffer from another one, but, unfortunately,

many people with celiac disease develop other autoimmune diseases at the same time. Some of these are lupus, rheumatoid arthritis, and even type I diabetes (the insulin-dependent kind). Yet, by far, the most common is an autoimmune thyroid condition called Hashimoto's thyroiditis. In this disease, your body makes antibodies against your own thyroid, and this can lead to severe fatigue, weight gain, cold hands and feet, and depression. In my case, this also lead to hair and eyelash loss. This was devastating for me, and it took a long time in my case to connect this problem to my celiac disease. My doctor says up to 15% of his celiac disease patients also have autoimmune thyroid disease. That is a lot, but in many celiacs, this is never diagnosed.

4. Cancer. The most common cancer associated with celiac disease is non-Hodgkin's lymphoma.

5. Infertility. This is perhaps the most common, but least discussed problem associated with celiac disease in both men and women. I recently read that the risk of spontaneous abortion in women with celiac disease is almost nine times higher than in healthy women. This may be what led to the loss of my pregnancy.

6. Dental defects, including enamel defects and teeth not coming in or coming in malformed.

7. Canker sores.

8. Dermatitis herpetiformis, a severe skin rash.

So this is what you are dealing with. It's not pretty, and it's not easy, despite what other people or books or doctors might tell you. I'm not going to degrade you by being some kind of rah-rah cheerleader telling you it's all going to be fine. It's not! Celiac is a disease that does not get better. It sucks that you have to have this disease. But you can move forward with your life, on one condition: You must stay far away from *all* gluten-containing products *for the rest of your life*. There is no cheating! *Ever!*

If You Haven't Been Diagnosed Yet

Some of you may suspect you have celiac disease, but you don't know for sure. Maybe you haven't asked for a test, or maybe you have but your doctor didn't want to give you the test. Or maybe you got a test, but the doctor said it was negative and you don't have celiac disease.

It is not that simple.

First of all, you should know about how doctors test for celiac disease. (Dr. Fratellone has graciously checked this information over to make sure it is correct.) First, you will get a blood test that checks your antibodies to the gluten protein in your blood. If you have already been eating a gluten-free diet, the blood test could be negative, even if you have celiac disease. For this reason, *you must be eating gluten when you get tested for celiac disease.* If you want to get the test, don't go gluten-free first.

The most sensitive antibody tests for the diagnosis of celiac disease are in the IgA class of antibodies, and there are three available tests for these:

1. Antigliadin antibodies

2. Connective tissue antibodies (these include antireticulin and anti-endomysial, or IgA EM)

3. Tissue antibodies (these include transglutaminase, or IgA tTG)

Most doctors, but not all, check the anti-gliadin antibodies, but this test is *no longer considered sensitive or specific enough to be used as the sole diagnosis of celiac disease.* Even so, this was the first and only antibody IgA test I had. I do not recall ever having the antireticulin antibody test, even though doctors now know that the endomysial IgA antibodies (IgA EM) are highly specific for celiac disease. This test can approach 100% accuracy.

If you have an unusually high level of any of these antibodies, then your doctor will want to do an intestinal biopsy, also called an endoscopy, to confirm that the villi in your small intestine have actually been damaged. The biopsy is a necessary part of the diagnosis. Dr. Fratellone says the biopsy of the small intestine still remains the gold standard for diagnosing celiac disease, and always should be done if the suspicion is high. Biopsy confirmation is crucial. This is a lifelong disease, and it can result in a high-cost change to dietary lifestyle, so you need to know the truth. Research suggests that the endoscopy should include four to six biopsy specimens, to be sure to check multiple areas for damage. This is why the blood test alone will not be enough to diagnose you.

But what if the blood test is negative? *You could still have celiac disease.* If the gliadin antibody is negative, get the other two serologic tests. If all three serologic tests discussed above are negative, still get the four to six biopsy samples. There are pitfalls in diagnosing any disease. In a celiac diagnosis, the failure to diagnose is in the hands of the doctor examining the biopsy specimen. There can be both under- and over-interpretation of the villous atrophy. Maybe the specimen was poor, or maybe the doctor didn't biopsy enough areas. Every test has a risk of error. Also, it's possible that atrophy of the villi could be caused by some other disease. It's never simple or straightforward—this is the challenge of diagnosis! What I do understand is why my doctor always says, "The gut is the gateway to all disease." It's so true.

There is an exception to the endoscopy rule. If you have the skin rash Dermatitis Herpetiformis (DH), and your blood tests are positive, you won't need an endoscopy, but you will need a skin biopsy. If the biopsy shows that your rash is DH, then you can be diagnosed with celiac disease.

Another good thing to know is that there is a genetic component to celiac disease and your doctor can test for this, too. This wasn't done until much later in my case, but celiac is an HLA-associated disease. That means it is associated with the HLA genes. The two genes most likely to be linked to celiac disease are the HLA-DQ2 and the HLA-DQ8 genes, and a blood test can determine whether you have these. HLA-DQ2 is present in 95% of those with celiac disease, and the remainder of those people have the HLA-DQ8 gene. The presence of these genes doesn't mean you have celiac disease or will get it, but means you could get it. The absence of these genes means you probably do not have celiac disease, so it's very helpful to know this information.

Beyond direct tests for celiac disease, there are other tests your doctor may order to check for signs of conditions that often occur with or because of celiac disease. You might get a complete blood count (CBC) to test for anemia, and other tests to check your mineral and electrolyte balance, your cholesterol and triglyceride levels, your thyroid hormones, and your bone density.

So you have it or you don't, right? Well, not so fast. Just to make matters more confusing, there is something called gluten intolerance. This is when your blood test does not suggest celiac disease, but you definitely have symptoms after eating gluten that go away when you stop eating gluten. If this is you, then you will feel much better on a strictly gluten-free diet. You might not be having the intestinal damage and severe health effects that a celiac has, and you might not have an autoimmune disease, but gluten could still be compromising your quality of life. Many, many people are "cured" of chronic fatigue, IBS, and other stomach issues, and low energy when they give up gluten. It's harder not to have that diagnosis in hand when dealing with doctors (and insurance companies), but you know what you know about your own body, and if you know you can't have gluten, then don't have gluten and don't let anyone convince you to compromise your health just because a doctor didn't pronounce you a celiac.

The diagnosis of celiac disease sounds straightforward, and yet it still takes the average person eight to ten years or more to get a diagnosis. Some researchers believe that up to 90% of those with celiac disease don't know they have it because they are either undiagnosed or misdiagnosed. If you are suffering and you don't know why, and if my story sounds familiar, then this could be you! You could be one of those 90% who are undiagnosed or misdiagnosed. The rate of celiac disease is probably a lot higher than the numbers say right now, so if you aren't getting anywhere with your health problems, ask your doctor to be tested.

And if your doctor doesn't think you need it? Insist on it. You don't have to be aggressive or rude. Just say something like, "I would just really like to know for sure that I don't have this disease. Please do the test." If it's positive, then you know. If it's not, then you still might have it and you have to keep searching. You might also have to redo the test. There is some evidence that there are a lot of false negatives in celiac blood tests. Even the endoscopy can be a false negative if they don't biopsy multiple spots in the small intestine, because the villi could be damaged in one part and not in another. These tests are not 100% accurate, and many people have only been diagnosed after multiple tests, so just know the test isn't everything. Much depends, among other things, on the skill of the doctor performing the endoscopy and the tech reading the blood work.

Trying to get a diagnosis is difficult, even excruciating, but don't be afraid to get online, join a celiac forum, ask questions, and do your own research. If you don't advocate for your own health and seek as much knowledge as you can find, then you're never going to feel better. Ask questions of your doctor. Don't come in and say you know you have celiac disease because you read it on the Internet (doctors hate that), but do explain that you are still not feeling well and you would really like to know. You have a right to know, and you have a right to feel better. Trust your instincts and get the test.

If You Have Been Diagnosed

A lot of the literature says that with strict adherence to a gluten-free diet, you will start to feel better in a few days and your villi will be totally healed in six months. Your doctor probably told you to "just" stop eating gluten, and you'll be fine.

Well, some people are lucky enough to have that experience, but I know many, many people who take longer to feel quite a bit better—up to a year to a year and a half, depending on how severe your case is and how damaged your villi are at the moment you give up gluten. Remember the detox I've been talking about? You have to contend with that. Gluten is addictive, and as it exits your system, you are probably going to feel a lot worse before you feel better. You can have major weird symptoms that I can't even guess at because everyone is different, but it's all part of the clearing out. Once you're free of it and you're not getting anymore gluten, the healing can begin, but the detox can take weeks or months.

You also have to contend with hidden gluten that can seem like it is *everywhere*. If you do "get glutened" (accidentally have some gluten), you can be laid out flat since you've been exposed to more damage that will have to be repaired. Even a tiny bit of gluten (an eighth of a teaspoon) can further damage your small intestine and make you feel like you're going to die. This still happens to me, after all these years and everything I've learned, because it's so hard to avoid gluten, and even products labeled "gluten-free" can still contain small amounts of gluten—legally! (I'll talk more about this in a later chapter.)

Then there is something called *refractory celiac disease,* which means that your celiac disease does not improve on a gluten-free diet. This is uncommon but it happens (generally, more than 90% of people who have been diagnosed improve with a gluten-free diet). Usually, celiac disease that doesn't improve is due to some unknown hidden source of gluten in the diet, but sometimes it's not. It's a wily and devious disease. Some people feel almost normal after a few months going gluten-free, and can stay feeling pretty good as long as they never consume even a little gluten (as I've said, this is easier said than done). Others will suffer health issues throughout their lives. It's just the reality.

But I don't want to discourage you. There is hope. If you've got that diagnosis, then you are headed in the right direction. You've gotten over a *major hurdle*. Just don't be fooled. You have an autoimmune disease, and that's never going to go away. I was told that I would feel much better as soon as I stopped eating gluten. *Wrong*. I also remember how sad, disgusted, depressed, and irate I was that it wasn't so simple and that I wasn't told the truth. I wondered if there was something wrong with me because I felt worse rather than better after my diagnosis. Nobody really told me about the detox period. There was so much I didn't know.

Now I know that I wasn't some kind of failure because I didn't recover as quickly as Ms. X or Mr. Y. I was me, and that's just the way it worked for me. Now I know that many other people share the same feelings of frustration for not recovering according to the schedule the doctor or some book says is possible. Eating a clean diet will make you feel better, but it does not cure you. You have to manage this disease constantly, and sometimes you will make mistakes, eat the wrong thing, push yourself too hard, or just wake up feeling like crap for no apparent reason. Don't be discouraged if giving up gluten doesn't completely cure you within a week. It won't ever cure you, and anyone who tells you it will is trying to sell you something.

Here's the real truth: celiac disease needs your constant attention. Damage to your health from malnutrition might have caused problems that will hang around for most of your life. (I still get neuropathy symptoms, joint pain, headaches, and skin issues.) You will live with it every day for the rest of your life, but it doesn't have to be a death sentence. A gluten-free diet *is* mandatory, that part is completely and totally true, but in no way will it solve all your problems. You have to take away what's hurting you, *but* you also have to figure out how to give your body what it hasn't been getting.

And here's the good news: Living gluten-free, healing your body, nourishing and taking care of yourself so you can start feeling better *is entirely possible.* It's challenging, but you can do it. You have to do it, if you want to start living again.

About Your Doctor

Choosing a good doctor is challenging for celiacs because you need two things: genuine celiac expertise and a compassionate personality. Unfortunately, there aren't too many doctors with both, but they are out there. You might just have to search for a bit and you might have to go through a few doctors before you land on the right one. A doctor who doesn't know enough about celiac disease is likely to miss issues, not understand that issues are related to celiac disease, or misdiagnose you. A doctor who isn't compassionate and who doesn't actually listen to you is more likely to misdiagnose you as well, and may also label you a hypochondriac or a mental patient. To help determine whether your doctor will be right for you as you navigate this disease, ask a few questions, which my own doctor suggested:

1. Have you diagnosed and treated many people with celiac disease? (A knowledgeable doctor will have experience with this disease.)

2. Do you do blood testing for celiac antibodies? Which tests will you do? (You want a doctor who will do all three types of blood tests, as well as the genetic test, or who will be willing to do them if you request them.)

3. Do you test for food allergies? (Not all doctors believe this is useful, but it can be a valuable way to uncover additional allergies and sensitivities, which are common in people with celiac disease.)

4. Is there a possibility that my nerve/neurologic symptoms could be related to my gut issues? (Obviously, the answer should be yes, with an explanation.)

5. Do I need a biopsy of my small intestine, regardless of my celiac blood test results? (Yes, you do.)

6. Who will discuss my treatment if I have celiac disease, and who will help me plan my diet? (Either your doctor should be the

person to do this, or should be ready to refer you to experienced people who can help you with lifestyle issues.)

7. Could the pathology results of my biopsy be wrong? (A good doctor will admit this possibility and be willing to work with you if you get a negative result that doesn't seem right.)

8. Does celiac disease occur in families? My grandmother had these symptoms and died of non-Hodgkin's lymphoma. Am I at risk for this? (Of course you are, but your doctor should recognize and be willing to discuss this.)

9. Is my inability to get pregnant/are my miscarriages related to my celiac disease? (This is quite well established, and your doctor should talk to you about this if it has been a problem for you.)

10. What are other symptoms in addition to "gut" or stomach problems that I might expect? (Your doctor should be able to give you information similar to what you find in this chapter.)

The problem is that a lot of the doctors out there don't listen to you, or they already have it in their head what's wrong with you before they actually know. You need a doctor who will really listen to what you're saying and take the time to do the tests you need. You don't need a doctor who will say, "Just stop eating gluten and see me in a year." You need a doctor who will hear you, not make you a case study or decide you are exactly like the six other patients that kind of seem like you.

A good doctor will ask you what you are eating, what vitamins you are taking, and will tell you what you should be doing to get healthy, not just stop the damage. Look for someone who looks at you as a whole, and at your body as a whole. You are not part of a group. You are an individual. Go with your gut and your instinct about your own health. If you aren't being heard, you have the right to look for a different doctor—and when you find one, you will discover that they are worth their weight in gold.

17

after diagnosis: what next?

*B*eing diagnosed with celiac disease is daunting in so many ways. Maybe you will be glad, or feel relieved. But then the questions start. You will have many, many questions about your health, and every time something goes wrong, you will wonder if it's related to celiac disease. (Chances are, it will be.)

You might also be angry. Crying, screaming, feeling like wailing "Why me!" is all okay. I feel like people always try to look at the bright side of situations, and while this is great and can be quite useful, you also *must* be allowed to feel your feelings first, without thinking you have to edit yourself or put a brave face on. You need to be kind to yourself, and that might involve letting yourself get angry so you can get it out of your system. You've come through a difficult time and you have a hard road ahead, so give yourself a break. If you want to be angry, be angry! If you want to be sad, be sad. If you want to mourn for your past life, before you knew you had an incurable disease, or for the days when you could eat cookies and bread and pasta without giving it a second thought (not knowing it was hurting you), then do that without shame. The simple fact is that this disease stinks and you are allowed to think so.

But there is another side to this: I also want you to recognize that your life is not over. You may never be "normal" again, the way you once thought of "normal," but you can find a new normal. There is a life out there for you that is perfectly normal, *for you.* You need to make a shift, and that can be painful, but once you do it, you can find peace again. Until then, however, life doesn't stop. You've got a major adjustment period ahead, and it will affect not just the foods you eat and the products you use, but everything about your life. It will affect your family, your friends, your schedule, and your social life. It will affect your work and your leisure time, and it will affect how you think about things on the most basic level. But let me repeat: Life isn't over. It's just going to change. A little bit or a lot, depending on you, but change is happening.

Your doctor may not tell you about the detox period, which may be mild for some and harsh for others—it was certainly harsh for me. Your body was used to limping along on gluten, and gluten is *addictive.* It releases opium-like chemicals in your body so you want to keep eating it. Giving it up is not only hard, but painful. Plus, your body is healing and you still aren't nourished enough, so when you shift the balance by getting rid of gluten, there will be physical protest. When my sister told me that she almost felt better eating gluten than she did not eating gluten, I understood that, and you might understand it, too. But don't give up! You have to get through the detox. Eventually, your brain will clear up, your stomach will settle, and you'll realize how people are supposed to feel when they are healthy. But you have to be patient. It's going to take some time to get there, and the best thing you can do for yourself is to nourish and support your body through this crisis.

You'll have an emotional adjustment, too. There's no going back to the way you believed you were before your diagnosis. And that's okay. In fact, it's good, because eventually, you're going to start feeling better. Not today, maybe not tomorrow, but it will happen, if you do what you need to do to help your body heal. This chapter will give you the tools you need.

So let's talk about that. What do you do now? The next order of business is to transform your kitchen into a safe haven. It's time to get the poison out.

Your Kitchen Makeover

It's time to get gluten out of your kitchen, completely. If you share a kitchen with gluten-eaters, you will need your own part of the kitchen. Ideally, you would have your own refrigerator, but this can be difficult in many situations. Maybe you can get a small one. If you are the cook in the house, then you can keep your kitchen gluten-free and let your family get their gluten on the outside. This is no time to be selfless. Your own kitchen should be the one place where you are guaranteed *no cross-contamination*. Remember, just 1/8 of a teaspoon of gluten-containing food can destroy the villi in your small intestine and make you very ill. If you live with your family, your life will be much easier if everyone goes gluten-free.

This isn't as difficult as it sounds. There are good gluten-free versions of things like bread and pasta that you can make for your kids, and there are plenty of great foods you can cook with no gluten. It's just that we're a very gluten-intensive society, so right now, you probably have a lot of gluten-containing foods in your kitchen. It's time for them to go.

Get a garbage bag, enlist some help if you can, and start purging. Here is what to toss (or give to a local food bank):

1. Anything containing **wheat**: bread, pasta, pizza crust, flour tortillas, bagels, English muffins, breakfast cereal, doughnuts, crackers, pretzels, matzo, cookies, muffins, cupcakes, cake—pretty much all snack foods, baked foods, and pastries, and most frozen meals, from diet frozen dinners to microwave burritos and frozen pizza.

This is probably going to be your biggest category. While you're at it, throw away the magnet on your refrigerator with the number of the pizza delivery guy. It's time to part ways.

2. Anything containing **barley**. Sorry, but that includes beer.

3. Anything containing **rye**.

4. Anything containing "cousins" of wheat: **einkorn, emmer, spelt, kamut,** and **triticale.**

5. Anything labeled "**multi-grain.**"

6. Anything containing **oats** or **oatmeal**. All conventional oats (unless certified gluten-free) are contaminated with gluten during processing.

7. Anything containing **wheat starch, wheat bran, wheat germ, cracked wheat,** or **hydrolyzed wheat protein.**

8. Anything containing **carrageenan**. Carrageenan doesn't contain gluten, but for people with compromised gut issues, it can cause gastrointestinal distress.

9. **Pet food**. If you handle it or your pet licks you after eating, this could affect you. Look for a gluten-free variety of pet food. Your pets don't need gluten. It's just a filler.

Other weird foods you wouldn't think would contain gluten, but do:

Breading and anything with breading, including **panko** and **cornmeal breading** (which usually has a base of wheat flour)

Brown rice syrup

Bouillon cubes

Candy and **chewing gum**, many types (like red licorice, malted milk balls, and many candy bars)

Canned baked beans

Canned soup and **soup packets**

Cheese spread or any **processed cheese**

Chocolate (some types may be gluten-free, but many types contain traces of wheat, so beware)

Chocolate syrup

Coloring, unnamed **flavoring agents, fillers, thickeners,** and **extenders,** including **malts, starches,** and **dextrates.** That includes anything containing: **dextrin** or any derivative like **maltodextrin** (usually from corn, but could be from wheat), **hydrolyzed plant protein (HPP), hydrolyzed vegetable protein (HVP), texturized vegetable protein (TVP).**

Creamed and **sauced foods**

Flavored tofu (plain tofu is okay if you can eat soy)

French fries (often dipped in batter before they are fried)

Fried foods (Even if they don't contain gluten, how do you know that the oil in which they were fried didn't first fry something in gluten?)

Frosting or **icing**

Gravy and **most sauces**

Ice cream and **frozen yogurt,** many flavors

Imitation crab sticks

Ketchup, mustard, and **mayonnaise**

Malt vinegar

Marinade

Nut and **snack mixes** with **seasoning**

Pickles

Rice mixes with **seasoning** and **sauce**

Salad dressing

Sausage and **cold cuts,** like **salami, bologna,** and **hot dogs**

Seasoned or **sauced frozen** or **canned vegetables**

Soup stock

Soy sauce

Sushi rice (usually contains wheat starch)

Syrup (pure, real maple syrup is okay for you, but not the fake stuff)

Tea bags (they are sometimes sealed with wheat starch!)

Tortilla chips, taco chips, or **flavored potato chips** with seasoning

Turkey if it is **self-basting** or **injected** with any **seasoning**

Veggie "meats" like **veggie burgers, veggie hot dogs,** and **veggie nuggets** (these often use wheat gluten because it has a chewy consistency that resembles meat)

Worcestershire sauce

If you aren't sure about something, read the label. If you still aren't sure, toss it. It's not worth the risk. Remember that "wheat-free" does *not* mean "gluten-free" because there are non-wheat sources of gluten. Wheat has gluten, but a lot of things have gluten that don't have wheat. If you want to get well and heal your villi so you can start digesting food and absorbing nutrients again, you can't play it fast and loose here. You've got to be strict and puritanical about this, even when people think you are being obnoxious or picky or overreacting. You are not overreacting when it comes to avoiding gluten. Let me repeat this because I want you to know it and believe it: *You cannot overreact when it comes to avoiding gluten.* Other people won't always understand, but you need to be an advocate for yourself so you can heal and feel well again. When in doubt, throw it out.

Now, what about your cooking tools and surfaces? Scrub everything down, and if you can, give away pots and pans and start fresh with cooking appliances and tools that have never touched gluten. If you can't do this right now, just clean them extremely well. Toasters are cheap, and I highly recommend getting rid of your toaster and buying a new one that will never touch gluten, because it's almost impossible to clean all the gluten out of a used toaster (if you're sharing a space with someone who eats gluten, keep two toasters). I also recommend a fresh set of baking equipment. Cookie sheets, baking pans, muffin tins, and wooden spoons are cheap at discount stores.

After this little exercise, you may find that your refrigerator and cupboards are pretty bare. That's what happened to me. I sat in my empty kitchen with the bare cupboards practically echoing and wondered what the heck I was going to eat. Just hold on, we'll get to that. But first, we have more work to do.

Your Bathroom Makeover

Drag out another garbage bag because we're not done purging yet. You don't want to eat gluten, but you don't want to put it on your skin, either, and a lot of personal products contain gluten, or *might* contain gluten. This can affect you seriously and severely. Five years after I went gluten-free, I was suffering from terrible burning on my scalp. Then I read the ingredients on my shampoo. Sure enough, it contained gluten. I switched to a gluten-free shampoo (I really like the Acure organic shampoo brand), and the burning completely disappeared.

There are some really high quality, gluten-free personal products, but one of my favorites is plain old coconut oil. It's a great moisturizer for the skin (unless you have an allergy to coconut).

Fortunately, more non-food products are now being labeled "gluten-free," but if you aren't sure, read the ingredients list for suspicious ingredients, and toss it. Products that may contain gluten include:

Baby powder
Bath salts
Body lotion
Body wash
Body, hand, and face lotion
Bubble bath
Conditioner

Cough drops
Cough syrup and cough drops
Lipstick, lip gloss, and lip balm
Makeup
Mouthwash
Oatmeal products (like oatmeal bath products or lotions for
    itchy skin)
Shampoo
Sunscreen/suntan lotion
Toothpaste
Vitamin and mineral supplements

Many types of medication, both prescription and over-the-counter (OTC). Your medication won't have a label so you will have to ask the pharmacist. Never rely on generic brands, which often contain gluten. You will have an easier time getting a straight answer about the gluten-containing status of a name-brand medication. Even if a medication didn't have gluten before, find out again if you see anything like "new and improved" or "better tasting" or "new formula." That means something has changed. Here are some of the ingredients in medications that could contain gluten because they definitely contain starch, and the source may not be identified:

Any starch derivative (other than corn, rice, potato, and tapioca, which are okay for you—if the starch is unnamed, don't risk it.)
Caramel coloring
Dextrate, dextrin, maltodextrin, or dextrimaltose
Sodium starch glycolate

Here are some words to watch for in personal products that could signal gluten:

Avena
Barley
Gliadin
Gluten
Grain
Hordeum
Oats
Secale
Triticum
Wheat

THE REST OF YOUR HOUSE

Many other household products can contain gluten. Sometimes it's obvious, if the ingredients say something like "wheat starch," but often, products don't have to contain ingredients, so always check with the company or look on the web site to be sure, for any product that will go in your mouth or on your skin. Consider that these household items may contain gluten:

Charcoal (the quick-light kind contains gluten and will
    contaminate any food grilled over it)
Cleaning products
Detergents
Envelopes, postage stamps, and stickers—the glue often
    contains gluten
Paint
Play-doh

Some people might quibble with these lists. They might say that this or that thing "probably doesn't" contain gluten, or even that they know it doesn't. How do they know? I'm not paranoid but I am careful, and when it comes to something processed in a factory where I don't know for sure the conditions, I'm suspicious—and I urge you to be suspicious, too. Just be on the alert. Keep your food and products pure and simple, with minimal ingredients, and you'll have the best chance of healing.

Stabilizing

Now that your home is safe for you, there are some things you can do to stabilize and nourish yourself. You haven't been getting the nutrition you need, and it's time to heal. The basics below are ones that worked for me, hands down. Of course, you should follow your own doctor's advice, but here's my list of basics that helped get me on the path to feeling better:

1. **Get your vitamin and mineral levels checked.** Ask your doctor to test your levels so you can get a good idea of where you are deficient. This can take a slew of blood work, but it's so worthwhile to know exactly what you need so you can take the supplements you need the most. You might be severely deficient in any number of things, but you won't know how your body is reacting until you test. Nobody wants to take a hundred pills every day; testing allows you to target your supplementation. Right now, you just want to take what you really need. Then, you can work up to more, when your gut has healed.

2. **Up your Vitamin D intake.** Most Americans, let alone most celiacs, are deficient in this important vitamin, and this is the number-one deficiency in celiacs. Vitamin D is produced in your small intestine, and since that is damaged, you may not have enough. You need vitamin D—it is essential for your bones, and a lack of sufficient vitamin D has been linked to depression, joint and muscle pain, chronic fatigue, skin pigmentation, and possibly even Alzheimer's disease! Most people who've just been diagnosed need to start replenishing it immediately.

The problem is, if you can barely digest food, you certainly can't digest horse pill-sized vitamins. I found that taking vitamins in liquid or powder form made it as easy as possible for my damaged digestive system to take in those nutrients. Consult with your doctor on what dosage is right for you.

You can also eat vitamin D-rich foods, like fish (especially herring, catfish, salmon, trout, halibut, sardines, and mackerel), fish liver oil, egg yolks (if you aren't allergic to eggs), and foods that are fortified with vitamin D (like some non-gluten grains and dairy products, although I recommend you avoid dairy products). However, since celiacs don't absorb nutrition very well, the very best way to get vitamin D is to take a liquid or powder supplement, at least until your levels are stabilized. Your doctor can do an easy test to check your levels whenever you go into the office.

You can also get vitamin D by putting your skin in the sun for about fifteen to twenty minutes per day without sunscreen, but the vitamin D from the sun isn't the same as the kind produced in the small intestine. Your body needs to convert it, and since all things nutrient related aren't working so great for you right now, you probably also need a supplement. In my case, I couldn't get vitamin D from the sun until I got back into balance. My body didn't know what to do with that vitamin D, and started attacking my skin. Remember, you have an autoimmune system so your body gets confused. You need to be gentle and do what works for you. **Cover your bases.** A gentle powder or liquid multivitamin and extra vitamin C for a more balanced immune system may also really help you, as long as it doesn't upset your stomach.

3. Add acidophilus. The bacterial balance in your gut is almost certainly off and a probiotics like acidophilus can help to correct the situation. Mega-doses of acidophilus helped me to replenish my gut with beneficial bacteria as I was healing. Your doctor may be able to recommend a good probiotic supplement, but in the meantime, you can just get some acidophilus. It won't hurt you.

4. Get some glutamine. This amino acid helps heal the intestinal lining. It's great if you have celiac disease, as well as for leaky gut syndrome. Find an easily digestible powder and take it according to the package recommendations. You can also make bone broth by boiling bones (any kind) for a few hours with onions, garlic, and a little sea salt, and drinking the broth.

5. Try UltraInflamX. This is a medical food formulated to provide specialized nutritional support (it's easily available online). I really benefited from this at first, when my entire digestive system was inflamed. It is a powder you use to make a smoothie. Try it for breakfast.

6. Boost your digestion with digestive enzyme supplements. These help you to digest your food better than you have been because they add the enzymes your intestine can't make when it is damaged, and that helps break down the food so the nutrients are more available to you. There are many types available in the supplement aisle, or your doctor may be able to recommend a particular brand.

7. Try sprouting. Help yourself along the road, especially in the early stages after diagnosis, by sprouting all the gluten-free grains, seeds, nuts, and beans that you eat. Sprouting eases these foods into your body by getting the enzymes going in the food and dissolving some of the toxins that naturally occur in these foods (plants manufacture these to protect themselves from predators). Sprouting will also help these foods to be less gaseous and bloating for you. You can sprout them yourself, or buy sprouted grain products (find these in health food stores). To do this at home, just put the amount of gluten-free grain, seeds, nuts, or beans you want to eat or need for a recipe into a glass jar and fill with clean water to cover them, plus about an inch or two more. Use any size jar or even a glass or Pyrex bowl. Cover the jar or bowl loosely with plastic wrap or a plate or saucer over the top and soak at room temperature for at least four hours, preferably twenty-four hours. It's easy to set up everything before you go to bed at night. The next evening, drain everything and lay it out on a towel to dry. The next morning, you can cook it or store your newly soaked nuts, seeds, grains, or beans until you need them. Drain the water and rinse well. The grains will get softer and mushier from soaking, and they will cook more quickly. If you like your nuts and seeds crunchy, dry them in the oven or in a food dehydrator after soaking.

As for beans and legumes (like black beans and lentils), I eat these now, but I don't recommend them when you are first diagnosed because they are always difficult to digest, even with soaking and sprouting. Once you are feeling better, they are a good source of nutrition, especially if you soak them first. After soaking, cook them with a bay leaf to decrease gas even further. I like to soak foods the day before I want to eat them. Just let them soak overnight, drain and rinse in the morning, and they are ready to go.

8. Know your allergies. Many people with digestive diseases are also extremely sensitive to other foods. Pay attention to how you feel after eating various foods, and if you react negatively, try cutting them out of your diet for a few weeks, then reintroducing them, to see if you notice a difference. It's best if you do this one at a time, so you can really pinpoint the source. Dairy is a common one, but soy and egg allergies are frequent, too. However, there are many uncommon allergies and intolerances, so there is no way to predict what yours will be. Some doctors will give you food allergy tests, but others say there is no solid evidence that these tests are accurate. Taking a food out of your diet and then reintroducing it after several weeks is the very best way to determine whether you are allergic or intolerant to that food. However, if you want to do a food allergy test to confirm what you think is a problem for you, this can help you be more motivated to keep that food out of your diet. Just be aware that your insurance probably won't cover the test, and they can be expensive.

9. Consider a rotation diet. Because I wasn't rotating my foods, I ate a few foods I thought were safe far too often, and now I am unable to eat eggs or almonds, and I can't even eat rice very often. Not everybody has the sensitivities I have, but I found great benefit in rotating my foods. When you are in a heightened sensitive state, as you are if you have an autoimmune disease, you can develop an intolerance simply by eating a food every day, even if it was safe for you before. If this sounds like you, try never eating the same food more than once every three or four days. Rotating your food also forces you to get more variety into your diet because you have to keep thinking of new things to eat, and that can help you to be better nourished, which you desperately need right now.

10. Go alkaline. Eating a diet full of alkaline-rich foods, like fruits and vegetables, is highly beneficial for anybody with a chronic disease. Eating a more alkaline diet can make a big difference in how you feel, how much inflammation is happening in your body, and how sensitive you are to your environment. At first, don't each too much raw because that's hard to digest. Gently cook greens, root vegetables, berries, and orchard fruits, or add them to smoothies. A lot of water is acidic, so you should test it. Squeezing a lemon into your water will make it even more alkaline—believe it or not, lemons are alkaline, not acidic. The more alkaline foods you get into your diet, the better you will feel. You can also test yourself to see how acidic or alkaline you are. You can buy inexpensive testing kits at health food stores. The best book about the alkaline diet, in my opinion, is *The pH Miracle*.

11. Get the Metal Out. You may not need to tackle this right away, but it's something to keep in mind as you get stronger. Get rid of heavy metals. Heavy metals, especially mercury, are highly toxic and kill the friendly bacteria in your gut, which can cause a cascade of other health and immune-related problems, making your celiac disease worse. Heavy metals bind to proteins, which the body then attacks, and that itself can lead to an autoimmune disorder. Heavy metals also increase free radicals and acidity in the body, leading to chronic inflammation, hormone issues, chronic fatigue, weight gain, thyroid issues, depression, nervous system issues, and more. Most of us have heavy metals, but if you have celiac disease or any other autoimmune disease, you want to reduce these as much as possible because your system is extra sensitive and easily damaged. Some supplements that can help gently detoxify your body from heavy metals: glutathione, cilantro, burdock, blue-green algae (also called chlorella), and selenium. Also, eat lots of onions and garlic, which contain many properties that can help to detoxify you.

Try some or all of these things, and see how you do. Now, let's talk about what you can eat!

18

relearning how to eat

When I was first diagnosed and learned everything I couldn't eat, I despaired. Everything I loved was off the list! It took me awhile, and a lot of experimenting, to figure out that there were many delicious foods I could still eat, and ways to eat that would best nourish and fortify me without making me ill. But how I ate at first was quite different than how I eat now. At first, you must be very gentle with yourself.

What to Eat When You Are First Diagnosed

Inflammation is a big problem with celiacs. The year before my diagnosis, my inflammation was insane. I was always bloated, with puffy pockets under my eyes, sinus infections, constant headaches, and brain fog. My stomach was bloated from all the digestive issues I was having.

Once I figured out that I had to stop aggravating my body and start healing it, things began to calm down. There were two products I used that really helped with this. UltraInflamX, by Metagenics, is a medical food for reducing inflammation and nourishing a damaged digestive system. Inflammacore, by Ortho Molecular Products, is a gut-healing drink in powder form containing L-glutamine along with anti-inflammatory herbs like turmeric and green tea extract (you can get both of these online at www.longevitynutritionals. com).

You already know what you can't eat, but you also have to remember that your digestive system is severely injured. If you break your leg, you can't just start walking around on it. You have to let it heal. You need to give your small intestine the same respect and provide an internal environment for your villi to re-grow. You also need to start correcting the many nutrient imbalances you probably suffer from right now.

So how do you do all that? You start with simple, gentle foods.

There are a lot of things I eat now, like salads and lentil soup, that I couldn't stomach when I was first diagnosed because my digestion wasn't ready. Cruciferous vegetables like broccoli and cabbage, especially raw, are pretty tough to digest. Also, beans and legumes (including soy). Right now, you need to stick to stomach-soothing foods that calm inflammation. Dr. Andrew Weil has a wonderful site, as well as many wonderful books about eating an anti-inflammatory diet. Of course, there will be things you cannot eat on his lists because he does not write for celiacs, but to learn what foods have anti-inflammatory properties, he is a great resource.

When I was first learning how to eat again, I made a lot of mistakes, but I had a few reliable standbys that I quickly learned wouldn't harm me. One was to take a plain piece of fresh salmon (not the kind frozen with seasoning) and wrap it in some parchment paper with some chopped, very light vegetables that break down easy, like summer squash and zucchini. Don't use any gaseous vegetables, for now. Add some olive oil, a few lemon wedges, roll it up in the parchment, and bake for ten or fifteen minutes at 375 degrees. It's that easy. Serve it over brown rice or potato—something nutritious, but not too high in fiber.

I also ate leafy greens, but only lightly wilted, never raw. You always hear about eating more raw vegetables, but if you've just been diagnosed, this is not for you. I always steamed my veggies well, or lightly wilted them, which makes them taste awesome. It also helps vegetables to be more digestible, without losing too many of the important nutrients and enzymes you need so desperately right now. Steam or sauté leafy greens with olive oil for just a couple of minutes, to make them easier on your stomach.

Also, chew with great care! Chew each bite of food twenty to twenty-five times. Digestion begins in the mouth. By chewing thoroughly, enzymes in your saliva will kick off the digestive process, making the food easier to digest, and making the nutrients more available for your delicate gut.

Some of the foods you shouldn't eat at first, you will be able to eat later, so be patient. Here is what a typical day looked like for me when I was first diagnosed.

Every morning, as soon as I woke up, I would have some warm water with a quarter of an organic lemon squeezed into it to help flush out my kidneys. Next, I made an InflamX shake. After that, I did some light stretching, to get my body ready for the day. Nothing strenuous.

Throughout the day, I ate very gentle foods—cooked root vegetables, soups, smoothies. No beans, no raw vegetables, no cruciferous vegetables like broccoli and cabbage, nothing gaseous or aggravating. This time is about letting your digestive system rest and heal. I also drank ginger and chamomile tea many times per day, throughout the day (see below for some ginger tea tips). **Peppermint tea** is a wonderful tea to help fight nausea, indigestion, and gas. I was often hungry in the beginning, but so afraid to eat anything because I didn't want to make myself sick. You'll find recipes for the gentle, soothing, and easy-to-make recipes I relied on heavily in those early days on pages 256, 257, 264 (Jennifer's Smoothie, Kill the Germs Tea, and Sweet Potato Fries).

Juices

Drinking fresh juice is a great alternative to always making your stomach break down hard pieces of raw veggies. It gives you the nutritional benefits of consuming raw produce while being much more easily absorbed and gentler on your digestive system. I recommend getting your own juicer, but a good blender can also do the trick. I strongly advise making your own juice at home because it's the easiest way to avoid cross-contamination.

Most juice places do lots of different veggie and fruit juice blends in the same machines, and some of those might contain sprouts and grasses that you need to avoid. Wheat and barley grasses are just two of the ingredients you need to watch out for. While it's said that wheat grass is safe because it's used at such an early stage in its development that gluten hasn't had a chance to form yet, I say, don't do it. Play it safe. I, along with a few other celiacs I know, have felt a little off after drinking juice made with machinery that had just processed wheat or barley grass. I'll say it again: Play it safe! Remember that it takes only 1/8 teaspoon of gluten to kill or damage intestinal villi, and six months to a year for them to heal.

These juices and infusions are great for detox:

1. **Fresh carrot juice** is loaded with vitamin A and good for treating constipation and other digestive issues. If the taste bothers you, you can offset it by adding some fresh apple juice and water.

2. **Fresh beet juice** isn't easy to get down, but it's great for liver detox and treating constipation. You should juice the entire beet because the leaves and roots carry tons of nutrients. Again, you can add some water and ice to help get this baby down. You can also try a carrot juice/beet juice combination, in whatever ratio tastes good to you.

3. **Aloe vera juice** is something you should make sure to get from a reputable health food store because you want the purest juice possible. It restores balance in your colon and promotes a decrease in inflammation. This juice is another one of my lifesavers, and I keep

it in my refrigerator at all times. When I'm feeling seriously in-flamed, I take one tablespoon and immediately start to feel relief.

What to Eat When You're Going Forward: Get in the Kitchen!

Once you've been gluten-free for a few months and you are feeling better and stronger, you can start experimenting with more foods, to see how you do. You may also be feeling more energetic, and, to me, that means more energy for cooking!

Even if you don't care for cooking, making your own food will give you a serious social advantage, not to mention a health advan-tage. When you want to eat with friends, invite them over. Who needs a restaurant? When you cook, you always know exactly what you are eating. Is it always easy to cook? Absolutely not. But you are going to be very glad you can do it when you begin to realize how little there is for you to eat out there in the world. When I have the energy, I would much rather have people over for an intimate din-ner party with homemade gluten-free food I made myself then to try to navigate a restaurant.

Safe food doesn't have to be gluten-free packaged food. In fact, the best food isn't packaged at all. There are many natural whole foods out there that have nothing to do with gluten. The basics for a gluten-free diet center around these categories of food:

1. **Vegetables**. All vegetables are gluten-free and should be a big part of your diet (just remember to go easy on the raw veggies when you are first diagnosed).

2. **Fruit**. Fruit is highly nutritious, nutrient dense, and perfect for when you crave something sweet. If your digestion is sensitive, try gently cooking orchard fruit and berries instead of eating them raw.

3. **Meat and seafood**, especially fish and poultry, which are easier to digest. Organic, wild-caught, grass-fed animal products are most likely to be the least reactive.

4. Gluten-free cereal grains. These include things like brown rice, quinoa, amaranth, buckwheat, and millet. You might not be familiar with some of these grains, but try them! You can find them in the natural foods section or gluten-free section of your store.

5. Tubers. These starchy roots are a good source of nutritious carbohydrates. They include things like sweet potatoes, white potatoes, arrowroot, and tapioca.

6. Legumes. When your digestive system has healed somewhat, you can introduce these nutrient-dense, protein-packed foods, including chickpeas, lentils, black beans, pinto beans, and white beans.

7. Nuts and seeds. Almonds, walnuts, sunflower seeds, pumpkin seeds, flax seeds, and chia seeds are all nutritious snack foods with healthy fat.

8. Natural sweeteners. I bake with things like real maple sugar, coconut sugar, date sugar, evaporated cane juice, real maple syrup, and honey. These are all gluten-free and contain some nutrition, which white sugar does not.

If it's a natural fresh fruit or vegetable, unseasoned meat or fish, or a gluten-free grain, you can eat it safely if you make it yourself. It only takes a few minutes to broil a piece of fish or chicken or make a salad. Cook sweet potatoes, brown rice or quinoa to have with it If you have more time, you can bake cookies, muffins, even bread. If you don't make it yourself, you never know what they've added to it.

You can have a nutritious and health-supportive diet using these foods, especially if you embrace cooking. Cooking has become an important outlet for me. It calms me down. On my very worst days, I can go into the bakery and cook and feel a little bit better. Sometimes, I go in at 5:00 in the morning, just to be quiet and alone and bake. I do this when I have a special order or a wedding. Even on days the bakery is closed, I'll go in and quietly bake something with no music and nothing else going on but the simplicity of baking exactly what I want to eat—not what's available, not what happens to be gluten-free on the menu or in the grocery store, but *exactly what I want.* It's a luxury we so seldom get—when you go out, it's about what they have that you can eat safely, so it's always about limits, never about freedom. To me, the bakery is about freedom.

Your own kitchen can be a sanctuary for you. If you're new to cooking, there are some great gluten-free cookbooks out there that will give you instructions for making a gluten-free version of pretty much any food you love and miss and long for (see the Resources section at the back of this book). Just focus on the best, purest ingredients, and invest your money in organic food because you don't need anything getting in the way of your healing.

A Note About Organics

If a food has a covering, like a banana or an avocado, organic may not be so crucial. If you can peel it, it's probably okay, but anything you eat whole, like a berry or a pepper, should be organic. The most important foods to buy organic because they are the most contaminated, or tend to be genetically modified (or both), are:

Apples

Beef

Bell peppers, sweet

Berries, all types but especially strawberries

Celery

Coffee

Collard greens

Corn Cucumbers

Dairy (including milk, cheese, and yogurt)

Grapes, all varieties

Hot peppers, like jalapenos

Kale

Nectarines, imported

Peaches

Peanuts and peanut butter

Potatoes

Rice

Spinach

Summer squash, including zucchini

Tomatoes, including cherry tomatoes, canned tomatoes, and tomato sauce

Always pay attention to anything that seems to cause a reaction. Could it have contained gluten? Or are you allergic or intolerant to it? Expand your dietary choices slowly and carefully, but also enjoy that you can eat more now, including delicious things like lentil soup, steamed broccoli, and more raw vegetables and fruits, like salads and apples.

What I Eat Now

Most of the things I eat for breakfast take a little time, but it is so important that you give yourself some time in the morning to wake up and get going. Your mornings should be *relaxing*. Some breakfast suggestions:

QUICK BREAKFASTS:

   1. Grapefruit (starting your day with lemon water and grapefruit is a great way to alkalize your body first thing in the morning)

   2. Quinoa or rice crackers with some nut butter or fresh jam (watch out for preservatives and other filler ingredients)

   3. Apple with nut butter

   4. Banana with nut butter

   5. A handful of blueberries and a handful of nuts

   6. Jennifer's Smoothie (recipe on page 257)

   7. Chia seed pudding, prepped the night before (recipe on page 258)

BREAKFASTS THAT TAKE A BIT MORE TIME, BUT ARE WORTH IT:

   1. A warm bowl of cooked quinoa or amaranth

   2. Quinoa porridge with fruit and nuts

   3. Gluten-free muffin or banana bread (recipe on page 261)

4. Hard-boiled eggs (if you aren't allergic to them—many people are and may not know it)

5. An omelette

6. Gluten-free pancakes. You can make pancakes out of buckwheat, or see my recipe for

7. Buckwheat Pancakes (page 262) or Pumpkin Hazelnut Chocolate Chip Pancakes (page 263)

For lunch, I often have something simple, like a little soup or a salad with some protein, and for dinner, I love to cook something really hearty and filling. I also like to snack throughout the day. Fruit, nuts, raw veggies, a gluten-free homemade baked treat—these are all good to bring to work with you or stick in your purse when you are on the run. Use any of the recipes in this book to make your other meals but also remember that many pure, natural food that don't require any cooking are naturally gluten-free: fruit, vegetables, gluten-free grains, and animal protein. The more processed it is, the more likely it might contain some gluten. The more natural it is, the less likely anything has been added that you don't know about, and the better your body will be able to digest and extract the nutrients. Have some homemade soup for a snack, or blend a quick smoothie made from greens and fruit.

It's also so important to take care of yourself during the day. Monitor your stress level. Stop and rest when you need to. Or just stop and take a few deep breaths. Try to stay calm, don't take on too much, and be good to yourself. It's not always easy—believe me, I know. Life is demanding. But if you crash and end up in bed for days, you won't be any good to anyone, least of all yourself.

Finally, if you love sweets like I do, please remember that **you** don't have to give them up. Just make them better for you. I've added some of the simple favorites from my bakery that can take you a long way. Not only are they delicious, but they are good for you and no one will care or even notice that they are gluten-free. See pages 256–270.

Going Out to Dinner

Finally, in a chapter about food, I need to address the fact that sometimes, we all just want to go to a nice restaurant, relax, eat good food, and go home without having to clean up a mess. When I was first diagnosed, I thought I could never go to a restaurant again, but I finally learned how to do it.

Some of the time, you actually might not want to eat at the restaurant. That goes against what I just said, but it's just easier when people want to go out and you want to go, too, and enjoy the company, but not deal with trying to find something safe to eat. My cardinal rule in these situations is to eat something at home first. This way, you don't risk making a mistake. You don't have to eat to go and have a good time with your friends. People may give you trouble about it, but you might as well get used to that. You don't have to like it, but it's good to have some prepared responses like, "Thanks, but I just ate. I'm here to enjoy the company," or "Trust me, you don't want me to eat this food." You don't need to be embarrassed or ashamed. Just be straightforward.

You and only you know and can say how you should or shouldn't or can or can't eat. End of story. It's nobody else's business, anyway. I know a lot of gluten-free books and web sites out there will give you lists of chains with gluten-free menus, but I'm going to tell you the opposite of what they say: don't do it. I don't need PF Chang's or Outback Steakhouse to write me angry letters—this is just my opinion: unless the restaurant has a totally dedicated gluten-free kitchen, or a serious tried-and-tested separate area of the kitchen, I just cannot recommend eating at that or any restaurant that doesn't adhere to strict guidelines about how to cook for celiacs. I just can't. If you were my dearest friend—as any celiac is to me now—I would tell you not to risk it.

A woman who has been a celiac a very long time, and is still quite ill, came into the bakery a couple of times. I asked her, "What do you eat?" She said she goes to this chain restaurant and that chain restaurant, eating out a lot. This could have a lot to do with why she isn't feeling well. She told me about all their gluten-free menus, but cross-contamination can happen so easily that most restaurants won't *guarantee* that their gluten-free entrees are truly gluten-free. Remember, it takes just 1/8 of a teaspoon of gluten-containing food or residue to seriously damage your villi. Better just to have a glass of wine and relax while everyone else eats. If you've eaten first, you won't be tempted.

That being said, there are two restaurants (in all of New York City) that I can go to and reliably not get sick, but I'm not going to name them because I never know when something might change and I don't want to lead you astray. You have to find out where you can go and who you can trust for yourself. You might be able to find a place or two where you live, and you can increase your odds by having a serious heart-to-heart with the owner and the chef. Here's what you do.

First, start with one of the small mom-and-pop restaurants, lo-cally owned. They are likely to be more flexible and to use fresher, more real ingredients. Then you need to sit down with them and look them in the eye and say: "Listen, I want to come to this restau-rant. I want to be your customer. But if I get any gluten in my food, even residue from something, I will be deathly ill. I will fall on your floor. I will puke in your bathroom. Do you understand and can you help me? Is there food you can make for me that does not touch any gluten food, or any surface that touches gluten food?"

And maybe they will help you. And maybe they won't. You can tell a lot by looking someone in the face, being very clear to them, and then using your intuition to determine whether they are lis-tening to you and whether or not they give a damn. When you find someone who does give a damn, who is willing to do what it takes to feed you, who wants to really try to keep you as a customer, then you can start developing a relationship. I just keep going back to those two restaurants I trust. They have my business and my loyalty.

I hope you have a better idea now of what to eat and what not to eat, how to start cooking, and how to take back some of your power. It's hard, but it's possible. This is part of your new life, so I hope you will embrace it. You can do this.

19

the invisible disease

Everyone has the right to eat how they choose, and taking part in the gluten-free fad is your right. You don't have to eat gluten, even if you could. I'm not telling you that gluten-free food is off limits for anyone.

But this presents a real and legitimate problem for celiacs. Our disease is invisible, so people don't quite believe it exists. It has become a joke in our society, but we can't afford to joke about it. It isn't funny to those of us who rely on gluten-free food to survive. We didn't choose it, and we suffer all the time because of it. And because of the fad, we suffer even more. "But you don't look sick," are words that are very hard to hear when you feel horrendous, and people judge you from the outside when the inside feels very different. Of course no one wants to look sick, but, unfortunately, people have a hard time believing in something they can't actually see.

How eating gluten-free became the butt of every comedian's jokes is beyond me. I've seen gluten-free diets and the people who follow them ridiculed in movies, on late-night talk shows and day-time talk shows, and in stand-up comedy routines. I understand that diet crazes are an easy target for jokes, but words spoken by influential people have consequences, even when the intent is laughter. If the public sees being gluten-free as a joke, a silly fad, or just a way to make money, or worse yet, something deserving of derision and disgust, that puts me and all other celiacs at a greater risk of gluten contamination when we go out to eat or purchase packaged food from a grocery store. I've said it before, but I'll say it again: only 1/8 teaspoon of gluten is all that's needed to make me, or anyone with celiac disease, incredibly ill. I've been "glutened" and been rendered unable to get out of bed for weeks. Then, there are all the restaurant owners and chefs and small product manufacturers who see this joking and derision or just the light-hearted attitude about gluten-free, and think they can take advantage of the trend and make some money on their products without actually making them truly, purely gluten-free.

Or think about the family member or friend or employer who doesn't understand this disease. They hear frivolous comments and laughter, and they think it's okay to make fun of someone who eats gluten-free, behind their backs or in front of their faces. Worse yet, they began to suspect that not only is gluten-avoidance not all that serious ("Oh come on, just eat the toppings off the pizza, stop being so much trouble!"), but they may also suspect that your excuses for not coming into work or cancelling plans or needing to rest aren't really valid, either. Maybe you're just lazy. Or a hypochondriac. Or crazy.

I could go on for days about why this seemingly harmless joking has a ripple effect, way beyond what I'm sure any on comedian ever considered when writing or making a joke about gluten. I'm not accusing anyone of being mean-spirited. I am simply asking people, from the bottom of my heart, to please, please stop the jokes. Even if you don't mean to harm, even if it really would get a good laugh, even if you would enjoy the knowing nods and mutual eye-rolling, please stop. This is not about hurt feelings. This is about people's lives.

This disease does not discriminate. It does not come in one size, it does not affect a certain race or age, nor is it one clearly defined package. It is not recognizable by one set list of symptoms. You cannot spot it walking down the street. You cannot see it with a stethoscope or diagnose it definitively with a blood test. You cannot look at someone and say, "You have symptoms x, y, and z. Therefore, you have celiac disease." It is elusive and maddening not only to you, but to the world around you. People are comfortable putting people into a category, doctors included, and when things don't make sense to them, *you* are the one who is "wrong," and you, unfortunately, will be the one to suffer. This is why I call it the invisible disease.

When you have an invisible disease, you deal with much of the suffering on your own, painfully and silently. Even if you explain in great detail what's wrong with you and how you feel, it can fall on deaf ears sometimes. Others can't see your stomach pain or muscle weakness or painful joints. They can't feel your panic attacks or depression or the mental anguish. They can't see a damaged small intestine, or a body so unable to absorb nutrients that every organ in your body is under attack and fighting for survival.

Sure, they can see a rash or if your hair and eyelashes and teeth are falling out, but they can chalk those up to all kinds of other issues. They can see the intense swelling and darkness under your eyes, even through thick makeup, but they will probably tell you, like they always tell me, that it's just age, or that you're just not getting enough sleep. I can't count how many people have asked me, "Are you tired?" or rudely told me, "You look exhausted." Yeah. Thanks. It's called *celiac disease.*

If someone just doesn't look very good, it's easier to blame them for an unhealthy lifestyle than it is to see this invisible disease. If someone is feeling anxious or panicked or irritable, it's easier to blame them for having a personality problem, a bad upbringing, or label them as "difficult," or crazy, than it is to see an invisible disease.

If someone can't go to work, or to school, or even out to meet a friend, or to a planned function, it's easier to roll your eyes and shrug it off, and call that person lazy, lame, flaky, or a loser than it is to see this invisible disease.

These are some of the labels we deal with, whether diagnosed yet or not. It's painful and hurtful, and it can destroy your relationships, your career, your reputation, your education, even your family. All because "you don't look sick"; and without evidence to support your complaints, your days out of work/school, missed engagements, and "flakiness" with friends, the outside world appear unforgiveable. Never mind that you are dealing with a *disease*—not an allergy, not a fad diet, not "craziness." It's a disease, and a serious one, and the sooner people are better educated about it the better and easier all of our lives will be.

What everyone needs to remember is that no one with celiac disease *chose* to have celiac disease.

Judgment

I've been judged by my appearance all my life—you probably have been, too. If you don't look sick, then good for you—but when someone judges you and your capabilities based on how you look, they are often going to get it wrong, especially in the case of a celiac. If how you look doesn't match how ill you are or how serious your disease is, then judgment isn't just insulting. It can be life-threatening.

You may also judge yourself. In fact, I'm sure you do. If you are dealing with horrible health issues, but you can't get a diagnosis, you may think you just need to change your attitude, or go on a different diet, or manage your stress better, or just do something differently because *it must be your fault.*

Then, once you do get diagnosed, you might judge yourself again. If you are eating gluten-free (or you think you are), but you still deal with horrible health, then you might decide that it's your fault again. You're a *bad celiac!*

With celiac disease, there is almost an attitude that those who suffer from it *deserve* the jokes and ridicule. People think those of us who cannot eat gluten are just being difficult or making a big deal out of a minor digestive issue. They think our demands and requirements are inconvenient and annoying. We are *too much trouble.* We are *overreacting.* A "reporter" once called me a "spoiled celebrity wanting attention" after my last job on the cop show.

Recently, a woman and her daughter came into the bakery from Albany. The young girl was seventeen, and had been in and out of the hospital. She wanted to come see me because she said my blog was the only place where she found someone really talking about the downside, the ugly side, and the blatant truth of this disease. She felt like I understood what she'd been through, and that's sometimes all someone needs: understanding. She had a horrible history of brain swelling and other extremely severe symptoms, but she wanted to go to college. She has finally managed it, but it's a constant battle. She gets tortured in her dorm room because when everyone has pizza, they think it's funny to try to make her eat it, or stuff it in her face. Another reason why jokes about celiac are just not funny, but actually dangerous.

The Truth

Many people get ecstatic when they hear that a popular doughnut company is coming out with a gluten-free donut, or when a chain restaurant adds gluten-free options to the menu, or when a giant company that makes a food they used to love gets on board with the trend and starts making a gluten-free line of snacks or frozen pizza or whatever it is. But here's the deal: no matter how much those snacks and treats make you feel "normal" or like you have your old life back, most of them are full of crappy ingredients—and they may not be truly gluten-free anyway. Those giant multinational companies that make gluten-free doughnuts and invest in gluten-free menus and packaged gluten-free food (every big company these days seems to have a gluten-free something) don't truly care about our health. Okay, maybe some of them do, and to them, a big *you are awesome* shout-out. Unfortunately, however, most of them don't, or they don't understand just how strict a product needs to be in order to be truly gluten-free and safe. They spend millions of dollars trying to convince you that they care about you, that they've given you a gluten-free cereal, or a gluten-free cookie, or a gluten-free muffin, or a gluten-free Friday night spaghetti dinner special because they understand. I say double check and triple check to make sure that you're getting exactly what you think you're getting.

I've researched the ingredients on packaged gluten products and I've peeked into the kitchens of restaurants that have gluten-free menus. There is an actual ingredient in one of those "we care about you" cereals that is disturbingly close to formaldehyde. *Really?* Look at some of those gluten-free product labels for yourself. Ask to see the restaurant kitchen and determine for yourself how "pure" their center for preparing gluten-free food really is. Ask questions. Be an informed consumer. Even be a pain in the ass. Then you'll see what's really going on. Just *please* be aware.

I know it's tough—especially if you have a kid with celiac, and your kid just wants to eat what everyone else is eating. But do you really want to put a bunch of fake, "healthy" ingredients into your just-healing body—or your kid's? "Where do I get better, more healthy products?" is a common question I get. And the answer is actually really easy. I always say: Default to naturally gluten-free foods. Fruits. Veggies. Gluten-free grains. But I know you want convenience foods, at least some of the time; we all do. There are some small companies who really do care, who produce nutrient-dense organic food in facilities that are truly gluten-free. But you have to look for them. Look online. Visit celiac forums and talk to the people who have already done the research. But do it yourself, too, because formulas are always changing and companies get sold to bigger companies. That's why I don't want to list anybody. I don't want a formula to change, and for you to get sick on my recommendation. But there are good people and there is good food out there, and new companies and products come out all the time. You can order it online, and they will send it right to your door. Three companies I trust to source quality products:

Shoporganic.com, for organic groceries, cleaning supplies, personal care items, and products for babies, kids, and pets. They also have special products for gluten-free, kosher, raw, vegan, and pale diets, and you can buy many items in bulk, from dried beans and coffee to nut butter, dried fruit, natural sweeteners, and spices.

Vitacost.com, for supplements, vitamins, food, home products, personal care products, and products for babies, kids, and pets. You can also buy herbs in bulk, gluten-free products, raw food, protein powder, kosher foods, vegan foods and products, and coffee, and tea.

Gluten-free Mall, at www.celiac.com/glutenFreeMall, for pretty much every gluten-free product.

In the spirit of doing something rather than merely complaining, I hope that I will soon secure my own Jennifer's Way facility that will be a dedicated gluten-free, dairy-free, peanut-free, soy-free, non-GMO, organic haven where I can make my healthy, safe products available to everyone (not just lucky New Yorkers who can come to my bakery).

The Gluten-Free Fad

A woman came into my bakery recently and asked me a question that a lot of people have asked me—in person, on my blog, or on the celiac forums: "Don't you think it's so much better now that there are a lot of gluten-free options out there?"

My answer: Absolutely, positively not. No, I do not think it's better. I think it's one hundred times worse, because now restaurants are confused, and food manufacturers are confused, and *everyone* is confused. They are confused because they can't tell the difference between the person who wants to go gluten-free to lose a few pounds, the person who thinks they should go gluten-free because some famous person is doing it, the person who does it because they have some vague notion that gluten is bad without even knowing why, or the person with celiac disease who can become seriously, seriously ill from eating even microscopic amounts of gluten. People who are gluten-free by choice won't get sick from having a gluten-free cookie that's been placed next to a conventional cookie in the pastry case; people who are gluten-free by choice can have the croutons removed from the salad, eat the salad, and not be ill for days. The sad fact is that because celiacs are now suddenly in the minority of people shunning gluten, businesses may think that something can be free of gluten, but doesn't *really* have to be totally gluten-free because it's not that important.

In fact, there is even a new Food and Drug Administration Gluten-Free Food Labeling Act that says a packaged food product that is labeled gluten-free must contain less than twenty parts per million (ppm) of gluten. First of all, the act is voluntary, meaning companies don't have to follow it. And even if they do, the requirement says that gluten-free products can contain twenty ppm of gluten. Not zero gluten.

In other words, gluten-free products *can contain gluten,* legally, according to the FDA.

Part of the problem is that the current gluten tests they use cannot detect anything below twenty ppm, so even if a product has zero gluten, there is no way to verify that. So until we get better technology, and until the government takes celiac disease more seriously, this is what we get. (And this is just one more reason to cook your own food at home!)

I believe that everybody has a right to eat what they want and not eat what they want. You don't like gluten? Don't eat it. But I just want that very large and increasing group of gluten-free by choice people to realize that they are hurting our small, significant group of gluten-free people who actually truly *need* gluten-free food to live—gluten-free and pure and safe. I can't tell you how many restaurant menus I've seen that list gluten-free this and gluten-free that, and GLUTEN-FREE MENU in big letters, but which then have a very tiny disclaimer, in very tiny letters, that says, "Not recommended for celiacs."

Really? *Really?* This is not okay at all. We *need* this food. We don't want it. We *need it to live.* We didn't choose to have celiac disease. And you're going to single it out and dangle it in front of us as something made for us, but then you're going to tell us that it's not made for us after all? It's not just cruel. It's dangerous, because people don't often notice those tiny letters at the bottom of the menu. What makes me sad about the whole thing? It all comes down to money. It's not about health or weight loss or any celebrity. People love fads, and so does big business. Fads are sources of revenue for a lot of businesses. I get it, everyone has to make a living, but at what cost? When enormous multi-million-dollar industries have to get in on the latest fad, that's expected, but it should never be at the expense of people's health! Should it? If you're going to use the gluten-free trend to draw customers in and make money, then take responsibility, do it right, and make it for *everyone,* even celiacs.

When Medication Can Make You Ill

There is a regular customer who comes into the bakery all the time, and, like many others, she comes in not just to eat, but also to talk to someone who understands. She confided in me that because of her celiac disease, she has developed a serious thyroid problem, and that even after being totally gluten-free for a year, she was still getting sicker and sicker.

Finally, I sent her to my doctor. He took her blood and it showed that she was still having gluten somewhere. He thought her gluten-free thyroid meds were suspect. He sent them to a lab to have them checked, and, sure enough, they came back containing a small percentage of gluten. Small, but it was enough to keep making her sick. She'd been taking them for a year, and she was even more ill than before she'd started taking them. She'd been poisoning herself with medication that was supposed to be healing her.

I am not telling you to stop taking medication prescribed by a doctor that you need, but saying that if you can possibly stay away from prescription medications, do it. Medication should be your last resort. If the first thing your doctor does is reach for the prescription pad, it's time to find a different doctor.

Sometimes, you need medication. If you have a serious infection, you need antibiotics. If you have certain other diseases or complications that only medication can resolve, you may have no choice. The problem is that because celiac disease causes so many symptoms that mimic other issues (or turn into other issues), a lot of celiacs are on a lot of medications, and a lot of them may contain gluten. A lot of them may also be unnecessary.

I can't tell you how many people I've talked to who pull out all their bottles of medications and pile them on the communal table in my bakery, and say: "Look what I have to take every single day!" It's insane. If you get yourself back to health, you won't need all that. Maybe you'll still need some of it, but I sincerely believe that nobody, *nobody* needs to take twenty-five pills every day. Once you know your issues and have gotten off gluten and dairy, talk to your doctor about reducing or eliminating your medications in a safe way. But if you have to, absolutely have to be on medication, you *cannot take the generic.*

This is a huge point of contention with insurance companies, not to mention pharmacists. I've had so many unpleasant conversations with pharmacists who either didn't know whether something had gluten, or insisted that it didn't when their sources were not, in my opinion, reliable enough to keep me from becoming ill.

The problem is, the insurance company wants to pay for a cheaper generic, rather than a brand drug (and some will only cover generics). But you don't want that. The brand will have a more reliable ingredient list and can better tell you for sure that the medication doesn't contain gluten. Generics are cheaper because they often contain cheap fillers—often made with gluten. I've spent hours on the phone with the insurance company, explaining to them that I can't have gluten, only to hear some version of, "Well, it says the generic doesn't have gluten, so we're not paying for the brand." And then you're stuck either risking becoming bedridden or shelling out $300 or more for a bottle of medicine. It's disgusting.

What can you do about it? Here's a fact: drug companies do have to disclose everything in their products, but they don't necessarily have to disclose them to *you*, and they won't always disclose everything accurately. Generic drugs, however, may not have to disclose everything.

Your first step is to be sure gluten isn't already disclosed. An over-the-counter medication supposedly has to list all its inactive ingredients on the package, but a prescription drug likely lists these in the package insert. If you get your medication from a pharmacist, however, you might have to ask for the package insert. Then you have to know what you are looking at. For example, a prescription won't say "gluten," but it might say "wheat starch."

You also might have to go through a lot of baffling text to find what you are looking for, unless your pharmacist is willing to point it out. But even then, beware. Formulas change. People make mistakes. Companies lie. The bottom line is that generics are more likely to contain gluten. (And if it's a supplement, be doubly on alert: supplements *don't have to disclose all their ingredients!* They can have so-called proprietary formulas that contain gluten, and you might never know.) Honestly, all I can suggest with supplements is to look for those labeled gluten-free, and research, research, research. Ask questions, talk to other celiacs, and stay vigilant. It will drive you crazy, but until the FDA passes and enforces a law that every-body needs to label everything, that's the only choice we have.

Truth in Labeling

Of course, labeling doesn't just affect medications, it affects food. I know there is much talk about GMOs (genetically modified organisms) these days. A lot of our food contains genetically modified components, and we have no idea how that is going to affect us. What really disturbs me is the recent pushback against labeling food that contains genetically modified organisms. Right now, you would not believe the amount of money enormous companies—companies you think are on your side, "natural companies"—are spending to stop GMO labeling because they don't want you to know there are GMOs in their products.

My question is, if GMOs aren't bad for you, which they say is the case, then why not label them? Why not put it on your product? I'll tell you why: because they know people are getting wise to it all, and they know people don't want GMOs in their food. We have no earthly idea what kind of effect genetically modified food is going to have on us, and we probably won't know for at least another genera-tion. There was a study done on laboratory rats that were given only GMO foods. They developed tumors twice the size of their entire bodies! Food companies are experimenting on us like a bunch of guinea pigs, and on our children, too.

This has to stop. I personally believe the tinkering with the food supply is exactly why we have suffered such a dramatic rise in autoim-mune diseases, allergies, autism, and other chronic diseases, like can-cer and heart disease, in recent years. Wheat has been tinkered with so much that it barely resembles its original form. The same goes for corn. Even if a food isn't genetically modified, it has been selectively bred for centuries, so it is far from its natural, original form. Crops are modified to grow quicker, and taste sweeter, and resist pests better, and stay fresher longer. It's no wonder our bodies are so confused.

We should have a choice, and we should be informed, celiac or no celiac. Maybe you don't think GMOs are so bad. Maybe you like what they do for your food, but even then, you have a right to know what you are eating. To have a real choice, we need all the information. This is about full disclosure, and when you have celiac disease, you need full disclosure, in every form, in every aspect of your life, with everything you put in your mouth or put on your skin. Your food, your medication, your face cream, your lip products, all of it.

This is a lot to digest—and none of this is meant to scare you in any way. It's just to inform you about some of the things we are up against. Knowledge is power, and the first step to change. Let's start with how people think about and treat those of us with celiac disease, because that simply must change. It's time to stop being complacent and sitting idly by.

Talk About It

Someone once gave me a book about going gluten-free, thinking I would relate to it or that it might help me. I remember reading the part that said (I am paraphrasing), "At a social event, don't talk about it. Be light. Bring your own chips and talk about your favorite sports teams." That's when I closed the book and threw it away.

I refuse to deny that I have a serious health problem. How will that help anybody else understand, or raise awareness for what celiacs have to endure? I'm not saying I'm going to go out and evangelize about being gluten-free to people who don't want to hear about it, but if it comes up in conversation that someone has been struggling, the way we have all struggled, then maybe something you say is going to click, and they'll say, "Wait a minute, that sounds like me."

I have to say I've probably had a hand in getting about fifty people diagnosed, just by talking about it openly. A friend of my mom's was diagnosed with Crohn's disease and had been on chemotherapy drugs for years. When my mom mentioned that her daughter had celiac disease and that Crohn's is very similar, the man got checked, and not only did he *not* have Crohn's disease, but he did have celiac disease. He'd been taking those chemo drugs unnecessarily, while he continued to eat gluten.

I've also noticed that women are more apt to talk about these things than men: their stomach, nerves, hair falling out. Men don't like to talk about their health. It's a very difficult disease for anyone, but men don't like to go to the doctor for whatever reason, and they certainly don't want to talk about stomach pain. So, to have a grown man, a tough, burly construction worker walk into my bakery and say to me in his very Italian New York accent, "Jennifer, when I read your blog and you talked about back pain, I thought maybe I should get checked for this disease." He'd been suffering from lower back pain for years. He'd been given anti-inflammatories, nerve relaxers, exercises, and nothing helped. When he read my blog about lower back pain due to my bowels being twisted and inflamed, he looked into it, and what do you know? He had celiac disease. He came in and thanked me. You could see it was difficult for him, but he was so grateful to know.

There have been plenty of others whom I've met along the way who literally have come to me and said, "The conversation we had that night changed my life, and I got a diagnosis," or "Thank goodness you told me about the link between celiac disease and diabetes because now I know I have both," or "I never knew that having MS/lupus/another autoimmune disease meant I could be sensitive to gluten and dairy, but, thanks to you, I cut them out and I'm feeling so much better." One woman came in the bakery, an older woman who had only been diagnosed a few years earlier, who was trying her best, but her doctor hadn't given her very much direction or clear instructions, nor had he emphasized to her how serious it was to be completely off gluten and dairy. At her last visit, the doctor told me that she looked like she might be developing lymphoma, and she was terrified. She came in for treats, but wound up crying and begging me for help. Of course, all I can do is give my non-medical opinion, but I suggested that she forget about dairy and perhaps find a new doctor who could give her better information. I sent her to Dr. Fratellone, and she has since written to me many times to tell me how wonderful she feels and how she has avoided cancer. And how she is completely off dairy.

You never know what power your words can have. To have all these people come back into my bakery to say *thank you* with tears in their eyes is huge.

So, I'm telling you, you can have an impact. Don't be afraid to talk about it. Helping other people will help *you* get over your feelings of helplessness. Believe me, I still have days where I feel helpless, and I am not negating any of your feelings, but take it and turn it around, and realize that your words are powerful.

You now *know something* because you have a diagnosis. Think about how you felt when you didn't have a diagnosis and take the social opportunities to educate. Not to stand in the middle of a party telling everybody about your years of diarrhea and constipation and throwing up and falling down. You're not going to do that. But you don't have to limit the conversation to your favorite sports teams, either. All you have to do is say, "Here's what I was going through, but when I learned what was wrong, here's what I did." You can change lives beyond your own.

20

finding *your* way

I've talked a lot about food and other aspects of having celiac disease and going gluten-free, but the truth is that having celiac disease affects every single part of your life—your family, your love life, your job, your social plans, your travel plans, even your mood and your attitude. The trick is to figure out how to live with it. In this chapter, I want to talk about your life beyond food. I want to tell you what I know about supplements, exercise, heavy metal toxicity, and all the little things you can do to feel better today. This is a chapter full of tools I hope you will use, to make your life better right now, to help you find your way. You've been through a lot, and you deserve information that will actually make a difference in your life. Here are tips I've picked up along the way that have helped me start to feel better, have more energy, and get along in the world more easily. It's never easy, but it can be easier.

Resting and Stress Management

Getting rest and keeping stress at bay is huge. Stress has an enormous impact on the immune system, and many studies have clearly linked lack of sleep with stress, and stress with autoimmune disease. It's a 1-2-3 punch.

Stress remains my biggest problem with my health. It will take me out every time. Sleep, true restful sleep, is so necessary because it gives the body time to heal and detox. Make sure sleep is a major priority for you, and you will feel noticeably better during the day. Don't watch TV or stare at any kind of screen within an hour of bedtime, to calm your brain and thoughts, and stay quiet and mellow in those last few hours. Then, go to bed early most of the time. Anything you might have done instead of sleeping is probably not as worthwhile as sleeping.

Also, consider meditating again before bed, to calm your mind and body in preparation for sleep. It's also a good idea, in the morning, to start your day out on a calm and peaceful note. Try it—it might change your life. Just sit quietly, with no distractions, and check in with yourself. Here's one simple method:

1. Get into a comfortable position, close your eyes, and just listen to your breath.

2. When a thought comes into your mind, or you start thinking of all the things you have to do, just come back to focusing on your breath.

3. Keep practicing! It's difficult at first, but the more you do it, the easier it gets, and the better you will find your brain working.

Meditation does wonders for your stress level and brain fog. With celiac disease, your insides are struggling all the time. This gives your mind, as well as your organs, a few minutes to just *be*. If you are having trouble getting started, silently thank your gut and heart and liver and pancreas and immune system for working so hard for you. Feel grateful. Gratitude is an instant calmer.

Family Matters

I am close to someone who pretends she is okay all the time, for her family. She takes chances with what she eats because she doesn't want to make the kids feel bad, and she doesn't want to bother her husband with the inconvenience of her disease. When she is practically fainting from fatigue, she refuses to take a moment for herself to lie down. She doesn't want to burden anyone. For this reason, she is ill more often than she has to be. Now she has been diagnosed with Hashimoto's disease as well as the celiac disease she has been denying. I've seen this firsthand, over and over again. I hear people apologizing all the time for their illness. I still catch myself doing it, and it's time to stop. A woman recently came into the bakery with her son. I was in the back, and I heard her ask, "Is Jennifer here?" I came up front, and she just stared at me, then she started to tremble. At first she couldn't speak. Then she started to cry. Her son looked absolutely humiliated, and I could tell this woman didn't normally express her feelings. It was very sad. We need to honor ourselves and our bodies, and you don't help anyone around you by lying about how you feel or hurting yourself so you don't inconvenience others. It robs your family of their mother, father, wife, husband, sister, or friend when you aren't yourself. Part of who you are is celiac. It's part of the package.

Having celiac disease isn't easy on anybody, but if your family and friends love you, and you don't keep your feelings from them by saying, "No, I'm alright" all the time, then they could be part of your healing rather than inadvertently making you worse. They don't mean to do it, but if they don't know what's really going on with you, they will. Is it easy on them? No. But your husband or wife or lover, as well as your children, would rather see you feeling good than feeling ill. They would rather have your energy and happiness than watch you keep pushing yourself into more pain, or suffering in silence, or just being too sick or anxious or depressed to be an active family member. How can you be there for them if you aren't even there for yourself?

It's okay to say, "I'm having a bad day today, do you mind going without me?" or even "I really need to take a nap right now. Can you all manage?" It's okay to do that. *You have a disease.* It's okay not to be okay.

But it's not okay to insist that you can still be "normal." You can't be. There is no more dangerous assumption for a celiac. Celiac disease will not go away if you pretend it isn't there. On the contrary, it will only get worse. So can we all stop trying to be normal, whatever that is, especially in front of the people who love us the most? Can we all agree to do that? Admit that you can't just dash into a store and grab something to eat, that you can't take off for a road trip without any thought, that you have to take extra care about where you're going and what you're doing, and how you're eating, and when you're sleeping, and what kind of stress you are under. Admit when you need to rest, when you really can't do one more thing. This is your reality now, and that's okay, unless you refuse to accept it.

The only way to be well is to face this head-on and understand what it is, and make plans for it. You have to get up every day and think about where you're going to be, and what you're going to do, and whether or not you'll be able to find clean, safe food. And if you think you might not be able to, then you need to pack a lunch for yourself, right along with the lunch you might have to pack every morning for your kids. Their health *depends on your health,* so you have to make yourself a priority.

As for your partner, in particular, whether it's a spouse or boyfriend or girlfriend, that person deserves some great appreciation because loving someone with celiac disease does inhibit life in some ways. You can't always be spontaneous and your partner has to be an understanding person. But people who really love you want to see you healthy.

And if this causes problems in your relationship? Then you need to work through it, or think seriously about your options. You didn't choose this, and you can't cure yourself, so if someone wants to be in your life, celiac disease has to be part of the relationship. You may not like that, but when everyone accepts it, you will feel a huge burden lifted from your shoulders. And then you can get on with more important things than hiding your symptoms or wasting energy telling everybody you're "just fine." I hope you never have to say that again.

If you are with someone who doesn't accept you and isn't understanding, the only thing I can say is that maybe you need to think about that relationship. I'm sure it causes you a lot of stress, and that's not good for you. But if you aren't honest with your partner, eventually resentment will build up on one of the ends, if not both. Or, you're going to get worse. If your partner or spouse doesn't want to live that way, you might have to be fine with that, but they should *always* respect the fact that you *need to live this way.* They don't have to understand it completely. In fact, they won't ever understand it completely because unless they have celiac disease, too, they simply can't.

You can't force people to understand, but do give them the chance to support you. You should absolutely discuss it and explain what you're dealing with because that also educates people, and you never know who you might help with your words. But with a spouse or partner, don't expect them to get it completely because that is impossible. What they can do is give you the support you need to take care of yourself. And if they won't? It's better to end a relationship in which neither party will compromise than it is to spend your life suffering needlessly.

As for kids, that's a whole other universe. I don't have children, so I'm not really qualified to say too much about it, but here's the bottom line: if your child has celiac disease, whether you do or not, there is no question about doing what you need to do to get that child healthy again. No question. You just do it. Your house is pure. Gluten is off the menu. It doesn't matter if other family members want to eat those things. They can do it on the outside. Your house is a safe zone, period. If you can get your child healthy before he or she reaches adulthood, you've given a huge gift and saved your child from years of anguish. So you do it, like a parent would do *anything* to rescue a child from suffering. If you need more support, there are many online forums and sites devoted to raising a child with celiac disease. I hope you will visit them. You'll learn a lot, and once you've got more experience, you can help other parents newly struggling with their questions.

My biggest tip: try to eat together, and eat the same foods. No matter how tired I am at the end of the day, I come home and cook for my boyfriend every single night, and I make things that are delicious for both of us. I always involve him in what I'm doing, and he loves eating the way I eat because I make it delicious and fun. If you have kids, get them involved in shopping, meal planning, and cooking, too. It's a great family activity, and you will be setting them up to be their own advocates in the future, with skills to feed themselves safely.

Dating with Celiac Disease

Maybe you're still in the market for a partner and you're wondering how you're going to get somebody onboard with you *and* your celiac disease. A lot of single women, and even teenagers, ask me, "What about dating?" Of course, when you have celiac, dating is a whole different bag of tricks. How do you explain to someone you just met and are supposed to be having a casual, fun, get-to-know-each-other dinner that you really can't eat anything and you really can't drink very much? And if that person goes to kiss you? "Sorry, you were just eating gluten, your kiss could send me to the bathroom for days." I remember going on one date and trying to explain, in my usual passionate way. We were at a restaurant, and I was talking about how I would need to order, and he said, "Well, maybe you shouldn't talk about it as much as you talk about it. Maybe you should just try and live your life and not discuss it all the time. Get your mind off it. Stop thinking about it constantly."

And I thought: Wow. Genius. I *wish* I could do that. What he didn't get is that every meal could potentially be going to harm you, so, unfortunately, you have to think about it every day, every meal, pretty much all the time. Not only do you have to think about it, but you have to feel it. All the time. It's tough, I'm not going to lie. I'm fortunate to be in a relationship right now with someone who is very understanding, but it took a long time to find him. You have to be so hyper-vigilant that if someone has been eating gluten and goes to kiss you, you have to say no. You can't just let it happen. You have to be strong and let it be known when you need something or when you can't do something, and that's not easy to do, especially when you're trying to make a good impression on someone new.

So, this is how I did it. Remember, this book, and my bakery, are called *Jennifer's Way* because this was the way I chose. It may not be for everyone. First of all, my boyfriend and I were friends for years prior to being together, so there was a comfort level with him that I didn't have with people I just met. That helped. But even with him, I was afraid to reveal everything right away. I think that's fine, for awhile. It's natural to be hesitant to show your vulnerability. God knows I have a problem with this!

But be honest. Tell the person you have celiac disease. You don't have to go into all the details about diarrhea, and constipation, and neuropathy, and your legs giving out, or whatever your symptoms are. Nobody wants to hear that stuff. But I'm not telling you to lie. Just because you don't go into the gory details doesn't mean you can't be honest and say, "Look, I have this disease, and sometimes I can't do things other people do, so I want you to understand that up front." I'm telling you to put your best foot forward, but not to accept a dinner date or a lunch date or some other situation that you know is going to create problems for you. Instead, simply say, "No, I have celiac disease, but let's meet up in the park and go for a walk, or get a glass of wine, or a potato vodka, or a juice, or a soda."

I also recommend knowing someone pretty well and trusting them before you give them too much of your personal history. If you give people too much, then the questions come rolling out, and they may be questions you don't want to answer, or comments that will sting. I think I've heard them all: That I don't eat because I'm on a diet, or I want to stay skinny, or I'm vain. That I don't eat this or that, so I must not know how to have fun. That I should just eat the topping off the pizza or scrape the breading off the chicken.

It's no way to live, so get to know the person for a few dates before you really go into it. Even then, you might have a hard time. Two of the girls working in my bakery right now are celiacs. One is a young girl trying to navigate the dating world. A guy dumped her because of it. He said, "You're just not fun. You don't want to go out." She was recently diagnosed and she's dealing with a lot. Sometimes, she doesn't feel good. She can't go to most restaurants and she can't be carefree. And that's devastating, especially when you are in your early twenties. That's why there are dating sites for celiacs— another target for jokes that totally miss the point.

Being with someone who has celiac disease can be really hard. You can try to understand and be supportive, but you can't feel what that person is feeling, and you can't actually know what it's like unless you have celiac disease, too. You can't help that person you love, or save her, or fix him, and you can't take the pain away. Some people can't deal with that for very long.

It is what it is. I really do hope that if you are celiac, or you think you might be, and you are dealing with this disease that people don't understand, that you will give them this book. Maybe they'll read it and gain a new perspective on what you are going through.

So, with dating, you may need to try a few times. The first few relationships might not work out. Early on, maybe three or four months after my diagnosis, I told the person I was seeing everything, and when it ended, he admitted that it wasn't fun to be with me. He said, "It's hard to have to be so careful." Damn right it is! That's when I realized I didn't want to be around him, either. I understand—it's okay. It *is* hard to have to be so careful, and everyone has a right to an opinion.

But you also have a right to say good-bye. You deserve someone who has patience and compassion for your situation, even though he or she will never completely understand.

Dealing with Friends

Unfortunately, even your closest friends may not get it. Will you start to see who your real friends are and aren't? Yes, I think you will. Celiac disease may cause you to lose some friends. I've found it very hard to maintain certain friendships. A few friends have been great and have tried to understand as much as possible. Some have seen me at my worst, and they get it a little more than the ones who haven't seen how bad things can get. But there are always those others who don't get it at all, no matter what they see.

When I was losing my eyelashes and hair, and my eyes were swelling shut, I remember saying to one of my girlfriends, "Do you see my eye starting to blow up? I can feel it. Do you see a rash?" I could actually feel the eyelashes coming out because my eyelid would tingle. I knew I was having an allergic reaction and I was frantically trying to figure out how to stop it. And I just wanted to be able to talk about it with a friend.

But this friend, who was a very old friend and knew all about my disease, just kept saying, "Oh Jennifer, it's age. You're just getting old. We all are."

Age? I was so offended by that. So, this is all vanity? This is just me being shallow because I want eyelashes? And it bothers me that I'm losing my hair and my eyelashes because it means I'm getting old and I don't look good anymore? Is that it? All I really wanted was for someone to listen to me and hear what I said. I didn't need her to fix it or justify it or explain it away, because nobody can explain it away. I just wanted a witness, because sometimes even I don't believe what's happening to me. I just wanted someone to listen and witness what was happening.

You don't have to lose friends with celiac disease, but you should definitely cultivate some new ones so you have people in your life who really, truly understand what you are going through. This is why I believe it is so important to reach out to the celiac community. We are all in the same boat, and we are all willing and wanting to express ourselves and help each other. If you are feeling isolated and alone, or even if you are just trying to figure out if you might have celiac disease, go on my blog at jennifersway.org. You will always find someone on there who will get it. *Always.*

Celiac Disease and Your Job

How celiac disease affects your job has a lot to do with what your job is. Some jobs are flexible, but getting sick frequently is going to be a problem at most jobs. As you know, I had a very hard time with this on my last job. Sometimes, the way employers handle someone who is frequently ill goes beyond a refusal to empathize. It can even be illegal. The Family and Medical Leave Act (FMLA) says employers with more than fifty employees must give you up to twelve weeks off in a twelve-month period if you are incapacitated by a serious health condition (or need to care for a family member with a serious health condition). However, there are a lot of ways employers can get around this law, including by proving that if you are gone too often, you are not eligible for the position.

It's a difficult subject. Celiac disease isn't on the list of conditions that qualify a person for Disability benefits (although some of the complications and associated conditions are, including extreme weight loss due to a "digestive disorder" and inflammatory bowel disease). There are ways to get around this too, but it can be complex and stressful, and you might need legal help.

For most celiacs, however, once gluten-free, symptoms are generally manageable except for flare-ups related to gluten-exposure or other issues caused by malnutrition. I've certainly been through periods where I couldn't work, but after almost 20 years of being an actress, I can name three times that I was out due to illness. Those with flexible, understanding employers are the lucky ones. The best thing I can tell you to do is to be completely open with your employer, explain the situation, explain that you sometimes get ill because of the disease, but that you are doing your best to manage it.

And that brings me to another very important point: *your* responsibility, as a celiac.

Being a Good Employee (with Celiac Disease)

I am now on the other side of the employer/employee situation because I employ two celiacs as bakers. They both used to work in regular bakeries and were sick constantly. They came to me because they love baking, but they want to be in a safe environment and be able to taste the food they are making. They are both so happy to be in a place where they can actually eat what they are baking, and feel good about what they are putting into the finished product.

But I can't say it hasn't been frustrating when they get sick and can't come in to work. One of them gets sick quite often. I understand, and I would like to think that I am a human being first and an employer second. This is what I hope I get from others, even though it hasn't happened very often. Does the job need to get done? Yes, it absolutely does. But do you need to be a human being first? I say yes.

But I do have an important requirement. The only thing I require from my celiac employees is that they must be taking care of themselves. If you're going to tell me that you went out to a carnival and the sign said "gluten-free zeppolis," and you thought, "Hey, that sounds like a great idea, I'm going to eat some of those," then I'm sorry, but I'm not interested that you got sick the next day. You still have to show up for work. If you are taking risks and chances, then you have to pay the price for that and I can't help you. It is your responsibility as an employee (not to mention your responsibility to yourself and your own health and well being) to nurture your health, take care of yourself, and not do stupid things like eating carnival food or anything else you're not sure about. If something happens by accident, that's one thing. If you're doing everything you can to be as healthy as you can be, then I will be understanding.

I strive to be healthy every day. I watch everything I eat. I do everything I can to get enough rest, I try to meditate every day, and I really work to keep stress at bay. And that's what I expect from my employees. It's what your boss has every right to expect from you. Not to be perfect, but to be diligent and vigilant about your health. If you want to have a job, then this is part of it. Full disclosure, and making sure you eat really clean. If you want people to understand, you have to meet them halfway.

Restorative Exercise

That first year after my diagnosis, I could barely exercise, but what I could do was take my bottle of Xanax and drag myself down to a yoga studio right under where I lived. They had a restorative yoga class, and I would get into a completely supported position with bolsters and blankets that let me relax while opening my chest, and I would just lie there and try to breathe. This was one of the few times I felt real relief, because my chest, gut, and pelvis could open and truly let go in that supportive position. It was such a relief to get air into the deeper places in my lungs, which was hard when I was walking around or sitting because I was so inflamed.

You can do this at home with yoga bolsters, or just with pillows and cushions. Prop yourself up with cushions under your hips, back, and chest, so you are reclined but still sitting upright, at least at a forty-five-degree angle, in a way that you don't have to hold any part of yourself up. Let your arms rest out to the sides on pillows, and cross your legs loosely with pillows under your knees. Then, let gravity take over. Relax and let your chest and pelvis fall open. A wonderful book to take a look at: *Yoga as Medicine,* by Timothy McCall, MD.

Once you start feeling better, you might want to try a gentle yoga class, or just start walking, at whatever pace you can, for just long enough that it feels rejuvenating and not exhausting. Work up from there, at your own pace. Exercise is good for you, but keeping stress low and your energy up are the most important things at first. Mild to moderate exercise will improve your energy, but pushing yourself too far will only deplete you. Stay tuned-in to how you feel and give your body what it needs.

Rebounding (jumping on a mini-trampoline) is another great exercise. It strengthens your muscles gently, improves your circulation, exercises your heart and lungs, helps your body detox, strengthens your organs…and it's fun! It's also extremely beneficial for your lymphatic system, which runs mostly vertically through your body, and helps balance and vitalize your immune system and detoxify your body of viruses, infections, heavy metals, and other waste, so you can continue to heal. Mini-trampolines are inexpensive and fold up for storage, so they won't take up a lot of room in your house, and jumping on them will remind you of when you were a kid.

About Your Attitude

You have been on a difficult path. You've suffered a lot, in a way totally unique to you. Nobody's experience exactly replicates yours, and sometimes you feel very alone. But now, you have knowledge you didn't have before because you are learning more about celiac disease and your own body every day.

Whether or not you know for sure that you have celiac disease right now, I'm betting that you are on a journey to feeling better. And once you've gotten off gluten (and I hope, dairy) and started to take care of yourself and listen to your body and give yourself what you need, things will begin turning around. You can start healing yourself *right now*, and you are the *only* one who can do this, so it's up to you. Speak up for yourself. Get what you need. Eat what will heal you, rather than hurt you. Be patient with yourself, and don't beat yourself up for not healing fast enough, or doing well enough, or "handling it." And, most importantly, remember that no matter how hard it is, how often people don't understand, how hurt you feel, you are not alone. Get online and find us. We're out there.

As I leave you to go about your life, I hope you will come back to this book, and my web site, often. For hope, for encouragement, and for ideas. You can trust me not to look on some non-existent bright side or make clever jokes. All I want is for you to know what you're dealing with so you can get on with your new normal. The truth will lead you down a better road, and I believe in the truth.

Finally, you need to honor how you feel. This disease can affect your mood, your brain chemistry, your outlook, everything about you. When I get down, I get mad at myself, but that's useless. Many times, a poor mood is an absolute physical response, and it's not your fault. Why make it worse for yourself by beating yourself up about it? I say this, even though I do it myself. We must be kinder to ourselves! I know, at least for me, when I start to balance my blood work and nutrients, and start taking my vitamin D regularly, my mood lifts. Things start to look bright, and it makes me realize just how dramatic an effect this disease can have on my mood. This still happens to me. For the last few months, I felt like I was wearing a thousand-pound, wet tarp on my spirit, my personality, and my outlook. It's been horrible. But all I had to do was start taking care of myself again, with vigilance, and that tarp began to roll off.

So, I hope you can go forward every day and just value how you feel, and let that be what it is. You don't have to ignore it or make a joke out of it. Just let it be. Just explain it, if you need to. Say, "I'm not having a great day, I'm not. I try my hardest, and right now, it's not good enough, and I'm having a bad day." And let it be.

I had a great acting teacher in school, and he used to say that when you're in a scene and you're nervous, and you're feeling a certain way, that if you try not to feel that way, if you try to feel another way, like how you think the character would feel, you throw everything off. You are not present when you try to feel something different than what you actually feel

I remember thinking how interesting this was, and I took that idea through life. When you're not focused on what you are doing in the moment, when you are too focused on trying to be some certain way, or not to be some certain way, then you miss the whole moment. You miss it all. I have stopped trying to be what I wanted to be or what I thought I should be. I have stopped trying to look like how I think I should look. I embrace what is. Some days, it's shitty. Some days, it's glorious. But every day, every moment, it is what it is.

If you know what you have, and you know who you are, and you respect how you feel, and you live in tune with your body, and you stand up for yourself and give yourself what you need, then even though today may be bad, the next day will be better.

I leave you with this final wish: that you live in the moment, not of what you believe the moment should be but of what it actually is. That you are who you are, and that you let yourself feel what you feel. That you find *your way*. This is how you will finally get to your new normal, no matter what disease you might have, and learn to live again.

Be Well,

Jennifer Esposito

recipes

Basic Recipes

Kill the Germs Tea

SERVES 1

I always make this tea when I am fighting off a cold virus or any other virus, or feel a sinus infection coming on. This is a great way to help your body heal naturally. Mānuka honey, made from the nectar of the mānuka tree grown in New Zealand and Australia, is known for its antibacterial and antimicrobial properties; if you can't find it, local honey may help you with allergies. The ginger and cayenne pepper open up your nasal passages, clear out mucus, and make you sweat out those nasty toxins. The recipe calls for just a dash of cayenne pepper, but I add up to ¼ teaspoon.

1-inch piece fresh ginger
Juice of 1 lemon
1 tablespoon Mānuka honey
1 dash cayenne pepper

Peel ginger and chop it into small pieces. Place ginger in a container (teapot or jar) and cover with boiling water. Let it steep for five minutes. Strain ginger and add lemon juice, honey, and cayenne pepper. Drink hot.

For a very basic fresh ginger tea that's a great stomach-soother, simply peel and chop a one-inch piece of ginger, put it in a pot with some water, and bring the water to a boil. Once the water has boiled, let the infusion simmer for a few minutes more. Strain out the ginger pieces and drink, adding lemon if you like. Drinking this has stopped me from taking so many trips to the hospital just by relieving my intense stomach upset.

Jennifer's Smoothie

- 1 cup water, hemp milk, or almond milk
- 1 banana
- 1 handful of blueberries, blackberries, or whatever berries you can find that are fresh and organic
- 1 heaping tablespoon of Total Vegan (a wonderful, rice-based 100% pure multivitamin and mineral protein powder with no gluten or soy)
- Liquid vitamin D and powdered vitamin C

Blend and sip. Yum!

Breakfast Recipes

Coconut Chia Seed Pudding   SERVES 4

Believe it or not, those same silly seeds that made the Chia Pets so popular in the 70s are a powerhouse of nutrition. Chia seeds are loaded with omega-3 fatty acids, which are used as the primary building blocks of every cell in your body. Chia seeds also have as many if not more antioxidants than blueberries! Other benefits include fiber, calcium, phosphorus, magnesium, copper, iron, and zinc to name a few. Chia seeds help stabilize your blood sugar levels. You will feel full longer due to the fact that they absorb so much water and have such a high fiber content.

You can add the seeds to salads and yogurts or make them into this insanely delicious pudding. This recipe makes a large bowl of pudding. I like to eat some in the morning, as a snack, add it to smoothies, and even add it to other recipes. Chia seeds have no flavor on their own, so will absorb the flavors of whatever you combine them with.

> 2 cups coconut milk (light or full-fat)
> 1 cup water
> ¾ cup unsweetened shredded coconut
> 1 cup almond or hemp milk (at room temperature)
> 2½ tablespoons maple syrup (add more if you prefer a sweeter taste)
> 1½ teaspoons cinnamon
> 1 teaspoon fresh nutmeg
> ½ teaspoon vanilla extract
> Pinch of salt
> ½ cup chia seeds

Combine coconut milk, water, and shredded coconut in a blender. Mix on high speed until creamy. Pour the mixture into bowl and set aside. In the same blender, add almond or hemp milk, maple syrup, cinnamon, nutmeg, vanilla, and salt. Mix together on high until creamy and pour into a large mixing bowl. Add chia seeds to the milk mixture and whisk briskly until the mixture thickens. When the consistency resembles pudding, add the coconut milk mixture and whisk a bit more. Cover the mixing bowl with plastic wrap and refrigerate for 30–40 minutes before serving.

Apple Ginger Breakfast Bar   SERVES 9

In my attempts at cutting out most allergens from my diet, I wanted to see what I could create using the fruits and groceries I had on hand. I came up with this amazing apple ginger breakfast bar. The recipe is really so simple and so quick, and so yummy, and so much better for you than processed, packaged bars. These bars will keep for about a week wrapped and stored in the fridge.

2 cups almond flour

½ cup sprouted, gluten-free granola cereal (I use Lydia's Organics Sprouted Cinnamon Cereal)

¼ cup arrowroot flour

¾ teaspoon baking soda

½ teaspoon cinnamon

¼ teaspoon salt

1 ripe banana

less than ¼ cup olive or grape-seed oil

1 teaspoon molasses

2 apples, peeled and diced

1 teaspoon minced fresh ginger

Preheat the oven to 350 degrees F. In a mixing bowl, combine almond flour, granola, arrowroot flour, baking soda, cinnamon, and salt. In a separate bowl, mash the banana, add the oil and molasses, and stir. Combine the wet and dry ingredients, and then mix in the apples and ginger. Spoon the batter into an 8x8" baking dish and spread evenly. Bake for 25–30 minutes (or less if using a bigger dish). Cut into bars.

Sweet Potato Scones

Maple sugar has antioxidant properties and you can sub it in equal amounts for regular sugar. If you can't find maple sugar, you can use coconut sugar, date sugar, or even brown sugar, but those have much lower antioxidant and nutrient values.

1 cup sweet potato puree (bake and mash a sweet potato, or use ½ of a
    15-ounce can sweet potato puree)
¾ cup rice milk (or milk of choice)
⅓ cup grape-seed oil
1 tablespoon fresh lemon juice
1½ cup almond flour
½ cup arrowroot starch
½ cup brown rice flour
½ cup quinoa flour
½ cup chopped pecans (optional)
⅓ cup maple sugar
2 tablespoons baking powder
1 teaspoon cinnamon
¾ teaspoon xanthan gum
½ teaspoon fresh dried vanilla (or 1 teaspoon liquid vanilla)
¼ teaspoon ground cloves
¼ teaspoon salt
⅓ cup maple syrup (for brushing on top of scones)

Preheat oven to 400 degrees F and line a baking sheet with parchment paper. Whisk together the sweet potato, rice milk, oil, and lemon juice (if using liquid vanilla, add here). In a separate bowl, combine almond flour, arrowroot starch, brown rice flour, quinoa flour, pecans (if you're using them), maple sugar, baking powder, cinnamon, xanthan gum, dried vanilla, cloves, and salt. Whisk out lumps. Add the wet ingredients to the dry and combine with a wooden spoon. Take a heaping tablespoon of batter and drop on the baking sheet. Place in the oven for about 15–17 minutes (longer if you want firm texture and/or slightly browned bottoms). After about 11 minutes, or when the tops of the scones get a bit firm, brush maple syrup over the tops and then continue to bake. These scones will keep in an airtight container or Ziploc bag for at least a couple of days, or up to a week in the refrigerator

Banana Muffins or Banana Bread

MAKES ABOUT 6 MUFFINS OR ONE TO TWO SMALL LOAVES

Banana makes these muffins or bread (depending on what you want to bake them in) moist and succulent. This is a great recipe to make for breakfast or for a quick snack to take with you.

1/4 cup brown rice flour

1/2 quinoa

1/2 cup sorghum flour

1/2 cup potato starch

1/4 arrowroot or tapioca starch

1 teaspoon baking powder

1 teaspoon baking soda

1 teaspoon Himalayan sea salt

3/4 teaspoon xanthan gum

1/2 cup maple sugar, coconut sugar, date sugar, or evaporated cane juice

1 teaspoon freshly ground vanilla bean seeds (or natural vanilla extract, if gluten free)

1 teaspoon nutmeg

1 teaspoon cinnamon

1 cup extremely ripe banana, mashed by hand

1/4 cup applesauce

1/3 cup olive oil, coconut oil, or grape-seed oil

3/4 cup milk of choice (like almond, rice, or coconut—look for milk without carrageenan, which is hard on people with digestive issues)

Optional: 1 cup any nuts or chocolate chips, or a combination of both.

Preheat the oven to 350 degrees F. Combine all the dry ingredients, whisk out any lumps, and set aside. In a mixing bowl or the bowl of a stand mixer, combine all the wet ingredients except for milk.

Beat the wet ingredients with a mixer until combined, then slowly add the dry ingredients a little at a time, alternating with a little milk. End with the dry ingredients and do not over-mix. Fold in the optional nuts and/or chocolate chips.

Place muffin cup wrappers in a muffin tin and fill each ¾ full of batter, or grease a loaf pan and dust with brown rice or sorghum flour and fill with batter.

Bake for about 25 minutes for muffins, or about 45 minutes for bread, or until a toothpick stuck into the center of a muffin or the loaf comes out clean. These muffins last up to a week in an airtight container in the refrigerator.

Buckwheat Teff Pancakes   SERVES 4-6

½ cup potato starch

½ cup buckwheat flour

½ cup teff flour

¼ cup brown rice flour

2 tablespoons baking powder

½ teaspoon salt

1 cup rice milk

½ cup water

⅓ cup unsweetened applesauce

2 tablespoons grapeseed oil

1 ½ teaspoon maple syrup

In a large bowl, whisk together all the dry ingredients. In another large bowl, whisk together all the wet ingredients. Add the wet ingredients to the dry ingredients a little at a time and mix until combined. You may need to add a little bit more water if the mix is thicker than you like it.

Put a griddle or skillet over medium heat and oil it or butter it with Earth Balance. Pour the batter onto the griddle to make pancakes in whatever size you like. Cook for about two minutes or until the underside is golden-brown. Flip and cook for about 1 minute. Serve hot with your favorite gluten-free toppings, like Earth Balance butter and real maple syrup or fresh fruit.

Pumpkin Hazelnut
Chocolate Chip Pancakes
SERVES 4-6

When people who can't eat gluten realize they can have pancakes again, it makes weekend mornings so much more fun! This recipe has great flavor and the chocolate chips give it that little hint of decadence. It's a great excuse for having chocolate in the morning. (Just be sure the chocolate chips you buy are gluten-free and dairy-free.)

- **1/2 cup sorghum flour**
- **1/4 cup brown rice flour**
- **1/4 cup hazelnut flour**
- **1/2 potato starch**
- **1/2 teaspoons Himalayan sea salt**
- **1/4 teaspoon xanthan gum**
- **1 teaspoon vanilla**
- **1 teaspoon cinnamon**
- **1/2 teaspoon fresh ground nutmeg**
- **1/3 cup puréed pumpkin**
- **2 tablespoon grape-seed oil**
- **1 1/2 tablespoons maple syrup**
- **1 cup rice milk**
- **1/2 cup water or less, depending on batter - how thick or thin you like pancakes; opt for the thicker**
- **Grape-seed oil or Earth Balance (non-dairy 'butter')**
- **Gluten-free, dairy-free chocolate chips (as many or few as you like)**

Combine all dry ingredients and then whisk out lumps. Mix together all wet ingredients except the water. Add the wet to the dry, mixing as you go. Add water and mix as you go, slowly and a bit at a time. If you like a thinner pancake, add more water. If you like thicker, add less. I recommend keeping batter not too thin, or they won't cook properly.

Sweet Potato Fries

SERVES 2-4

After I gave up gluten, I missed having something starchy to munch on. These are perfect. Turmeric is an anti-inflammatory, and sweet potatoes are high in vitamin B-6, beta-carotene, vitamins C and E, and the mineral manganese.

> **2 large or 4 small-to-medium sweet potatoes or yams**
> **1 tablespoon olive oil**
> **1 teaspoon sea salt**
> **½ teaspoon cinnamon (optional)**

Preheat the oven to 375 degrees F.

Peel the sweet potatoes and cut them into French-fry shapes. Put them in a bowl and toss with the olive oil, sea salt, and cinnamon (if using). Spread them out on one or two large baking sheets so the fries aren't touching. Bake until soft with crispy edges, about 45 minutes. Serve immediately.

Sesame Parsnip Fries

SERVES 2-4

What I love about this recipe is that it turns parsnips into exact replicas of the glorious fry.

Parsnips are rich in potassium and a good source of daily fiber. They also store very well, up to 2-3 weeks unwashed in the refrigerator (in a plastic bag). Although autumn is their peak season, they're available year-round, and it's best to choose ones that are moderate in size and well-shaped—not pitted or shriveled. Sunflower butter—ground up sunflower seeds—is the surprise ingredient here. It creates a savory, crunchy coating. Delicious!

> **2-3 medium-size parsnips**
> **3 tablespoons sunflower butter**
> **2½ tablespoons sesame seeds**
> **2 teaspoons organic olive oil**
> **½ teaspoon salt**

Preheat oven to 400 degrees and line a baking sheet with parchment paper. Clean parsnips and peel outer layer like a carrot. Cut parsnips into thin strips like fries. In a large bowl, combine sunflower butter, sesame seeds, olive oil, and salt. Add parsnips and mix with a spoon or your hands until the strips are coated. Place parsnips on the baking sheet and bake for 35–50 minutes, or until crispy and brown.

Hearty Veggie Soup   SERVES 4

This is an easy, no-fuss recipe. Add whatever veggies you like. The water you add should cover them, plus an additional two inches. You can also add gluten-free pasta or rice by making it separately, adding it to a bowl, and ladling the soup on top.

   1 onion
   1 clove garlic
   2 carrots
   2 celery stalks
   2 peppers
   2 potatoes
   6 cups water
   2 tablespoons Himalayan sea salt
   1 tablespoon pepper
   1 cup chopped greens (like kale or mustard greens)
   1 tablespoon olive oil
   1 cup gluten-free pasta (uncooked) or cooked rice (optional)

Chop onion and garlic and place in a large saucepot. Roughly chop carrots, celery, peppers, and potatoes. Add them to the pot and cover the vegetables with the water. Add salt and pepper, and turn the heat on to medium-low. After one hour, or when you can get a fork through the potatoes and carrots, add the greens and olive oil along with the pasta, if using. Cook for another 10 minutes. Add more salt and pepper to taste.

Mashed Butternut Squash
over Wild Salmon and Asparagus   **SERVES 2**

When you are dealing with this ever-changing autoimmune disease, taking a "day off" is a luxury you just don't have. And when you're busy, inflammation can creep up, indicating that something is off. Butternut squash is packed with vitamin A and full of antioxidants to support a healthy immune system and reduce chronic inflammation (it also helps support a healthy reproductive system). The omega-3 packed salmon is full of vitamin D, selenium, and other nutrients that control inflammation. To round it off, some detoxifying asparagus also helps reduce pain and inflammation. An easy, quick, nourishing dinner.

> **2 cups cubed butternut squash**
> **1½ pounds wild salmon (about 2 pieces, though you can double)**
> **½ cup olive oil, divided**
> **1 tablespoon chopped parsley**
> **A few sage leaves**
> **2 teaspoons fresh lemon juice, divided**
> **Sea salt and pepper to taste**
> **1 bunch asparagus**
> **2 tablespoons rice milk**

Preheat oven to 375 degrees. Place squash on a baking dish and bake for about 30 to 45 minutes or until tender. When squash is done, remove from oven and set aside. Place salmon in aluminum foil, skin side down. Sprinkle with 2 tablespoons of the olive oil, parsley, sage, 1 teaspoon of the lemon juice, salt, and pepper. Close the foil around the salmon and place in a baking dish. Bake for 15-20 minutes, or until the outside is pale pink/white-ish and the inside is still pink. The cooking time will depend on the thickness of your fillets. Check with a fork; inside should still be pink while outside is pale pink/white-ish.

Take another piece of foil and place the asparagus on it. Sprinkle asparagus with 1 tablespoon of olive oil, sea salt, and the remaining teaspoon lemon juice. Close the foil, place on a baking sheet, and bake for 30 minutes, or until tender. In the meantime, using a standing mixer or a hand mixer, combine squash with rice milk, olive oil, salt, and pepper. Whip until creamy. Place whipped squash on plate and top with cooked salmon and asparagus.

Spaghetti Squash, Kale, and Tomato   SERVES 4

This delicious recipe is so great that you won't miss spaghetti made with wheat. I like steaming the squash, but you can also roast it if you prefer.

1 medium spaghetti squash
½ onion, chopped
1½ cups cherry tomatoes
2 cups chopped kale
½ cup olive oil, divided
**⅓ cup Daiya non-dairy cheese alternative (or dairy cheese, if you prefer and can
    tolerate it)**
1½ teaspoons salt
Black pepper to taste

Bring a large pot of water to a boil and place a steamer tray inside. Carefully cut open the spaghetti squash and clean out its seeds. Place the squash halves on the steamer tray, cover the pot with a lid, and steam squash for 30-40 minutes, or until a fork is able to go through it.

While the squash is cooking, add 4 tablespoons of the olive oil to a pan over medium heat. Sauté onions until clear, then add cherry tomatoes. Add salt and pepper. When tomatoes start to get soft, squish some of them down to get the juices out, but leave some whole. Sauté for 10 minutes, stirring occasionally. Add kale and the remainder of the olive oil.

When the kale starts to cook down, which will take just a few minutes, lower heat to medium-low, to bring the mixture down to a simmer. When the squash is done and cool enough to handle, use a fork to scrape the flesh out of the skin in a downward motion to get spaghetti-like strands. Transfer all spaghetti squash into a bowl and combine the kale and tomato mixture.

Before serving, top with cheese, more salt and pepper to taste, and even some more olive oil, if you like.

Banana Cookies   **MAKES ABOUT 24 COOKIES**

Sometimes, you just want a cookie, and this is an easy recipe with delicious results. Keep them in your refrigerator. Kids love these.

- 1 cup almond flour
- 1 cup quinoa flour
- ¾ cup certified gluten-free oatmeal
- ½ cup maple sugar
- ¼ cup arrowroot flour
- 1 teaspoon salt
- ¾ teaspoon baking soda
- ½ teaspoon baking powder
- ½ teaspoon cinnamon
- 2 very ripe bananas
- ½ cup almond milk
- ¼ cup grape seed or canola oil
- ½ cup chopped walnuts (optional)

Preheat your oven to 400 degrees F and line a baking sheet with parchment paper. In a large mixing bowl, combine almond flour, quinoa flour, oatmeal, maple sugar, arrowroot flour, salt, baking soda, baking powder, and cinnamon. Make sure that there are no lumps. In a separate bowl, mash bananas with a fork and then add milk and oil. Combine until creamy. Add wet ingredients to dry, mix until combined, and then fold in the walnuts. Scoop out the mixture with a spoon and place on baking sheet. Bake for 13-16 minutes, depending on how soft you like your cookies.

Oatmeal Raisin Cookies   **MAKES ABOUT 36 COOKIES**

For this recipe, it is absolutely crucial to use certified gluten-free oats, because other oats contain gluten. I was able to have oats later in my journey, but not in the beginning, so you'll want to be sure you can tolerate oats before you make these—not everyone can. The duration of the baking depends on how crispy you like your cookie.

3 cups certified gluten-free oats (important that the packaged is marked as gluten-free!)

1 cup brown rice flour

½ cup maple sugar, date sugar, or coconut sugar

¼ cup arrowroot starch

¼ cup sorghum flour

1 teaspoon cinnamon

½ teaspoon baking powder

½ teaspoon baking soda

½ teaspoon salt

½ teaspoon xanthan gum

½ cup maple syrup

½ cup grape seed oil

⅓ cup applesauce (no sugar added)

¾ cup raisins

Preheat your oven to 375 degrees F and line a baking sheet with parchment paper. In a mixing bowl, combine the oats, brown rice flour, sugar, arrowroot starch, sorghum flour, cinnamon, baking powder, baking soda, salt, and xanthan gum. In a separate bowl, combine the maple syrup, grape-seed oil, and applesauce. Using a wooden spoon, slowly mix the wet ingredients into the dry a little bit at a time. When dough is thoroughly combined, add raisins. Place tablespoon-sized pieces of dough on the baking sheet and bake for 15-25 minutes. These cookies will last about a week stored in an airtight container in the refrigerator.

acknowledgments

I would like to say a special thank you to:

My family, for the journey that has made me who I am.

Louis, for the light you bring into my life every day.

Dr. Fratellone, for renewing my faith in doctors and dear friends.

Rick Byrd, for everything.

Frankie Beans, my 13-year-old constant, unwavering friend and companion.

Old friends who try their best to understand.

New friends in the celiac community who were the first to reach out to me and tell me I was not alone in this.

Celiac bloggers who write endlessly in search of answers, antidotes, recipes, and some laughter. I especially want to mention my friend Gluten Dude, who speaks with honesty, passion, and great wit.

To Eve, for all the help, advice, and expertise in getting this book done so beautifully, and for her constant ear.

All who have helped make this book a reality.

My staff at the bakery and loyal customers, who say thank you every day and make it all worthwhile.

Dr. Mendel, who finally diagnosed me and put a name to the struggle.

Finally thank you to God, the universe, for guiding me and giving me the unending strength to keep moving forward.

Love to you all!

resources

Gluten free baking and cooking books:

The Healthy Gluten Free Life by Tammy Credicott

The Allergen Free Bakers Handbook by Cybele Pascal

Against All Grain by Danielle Walker (she also has a good blog)

The Joy of Gluten-Free, Sugar-Free Baking by Peter Reinhart and Denene Wallace

Gluten-Free Girl and the Chef and *Gluten-Free Girl: How I Found the Food that Loved Me Back,* both by Shauna James Ahearn (she also has a great blog called Gluten-Free Girl)

Pure and Simple: Delicious Whole Natural Foods Cookbook, by Tami Benton

The Gluten-Free and Almond-Flour Cookbook by Elana Amsterdam (she also has a good blog)

Other books that I love for naturally gluten free recipes (although they are not dedicated gluten-free cookbooks, they are full of inspiration):

Happy Days with The Naked Chef, by Jamie Oliver

Home Made Winter or Summer Editions, by Yvette van Boven

Apples for Jam by Tessa Kiros

Other great books to have on your shelf:

Healing with Whole Foods: Asian Traditions and Modern Nutrition,
   by Paul Pitchford
Yoga as Medicine: A Yoga Journal Book, by Timothy McCall, MD
The PH Miracle, by Robert O. Young. This is the best book about
   the ph factor in the body and how important it all is.

Great blogs and web sites:

Against All Grain: www.againstallgrain.com
Gluten-Free Girl: www.glutenfreegirl.com
Gluten Dude: www.glutendude.com
Elana's Pantry: www.elanaspantry.com